Acquired Immune Deficiency Syndrome

CLINICAL INSIGHTS

PSYCHIATRIC IMPLICATIONS OF

Acquired Immune Deficiency Syndrome

Edited by
STUART E. NICHOLS, MD

Associate Chief, Medical and Psychiatric Services, Methadone Maintenance Treatment Program, Beth Israel Medical Center; and Senior Instructor in Psychiatry, Mt. Sinai School of Medicine, City University of New York

DAVID G. OSTROW, MD, PhD

Associate Professor, Departments of Psychiatry and Community Health/Preventive Medicine, Northwestern School of Medicine; Director, Office of AIDS Activity, Chicago Department of Health; and Director of Research, Howard Brown Memorial Clinic

AMERICAN PSYCHIATRIC PRESS, INC.
Washington, D.C.

Note: The authors have worked to ensure that all information in this book concerning drug dosages, schedules, and routes of administration is accurate at the time of publication and consistent with standards set by the U.S. Food and Drug Administration and the general medical community. As medical research and practice advance, however, therapeutic standards may change. For this reason and because human and mechanical errors sometimes occur, we recommend that readers follow the advice of a physician directly involved in their care or the care of a member of their family.

Library of Congress Cataloging in Publication Data

Main entry under title:

Psychiatric implications of acquired immune deficiency syndrome.

(Clinical insights monograph series)
1. Acquired immune deficiency syndrome—Psychological aspects. 2. Acquired immune deficiency syndrome—Social aspects. 3. Acquired immune deficiency syndrome—Patients—Mental health. 4. Acquired immune deficiency syndrome—Patients—Mental health services. I. Nichols, Stuart E. II. Ostrow, David G. III. Series: Clinical insights. [DNLM: 1. Acquired immunodeficiency syndrome—Psychology. WD 308 P974]
RC607.A26P79 1984 616.9 84-6187
ISBN 0-88048-063-7 (pbk.)

Printed in the U.S.A.

Contents

Contributors

Joseph Barbuto, MD
Fellow in Psychiatry, Memorial Sloan-Kettering Cancer Center; and Clinical Instructor in Psychiatry, Cornell University School of Medicine

Carolyn B. Britton, MD
Postdoctoral Research Scientist, Columbia College of Physicians and Surgeons, Columbia University

James W. Dilley, MD
Assistant Clinical Professor of Psychiatry, University of California School of Medicine, San Francisco General Hospital

Roger W. Enlow, MD
Director, Office of Lesbian and Gay Health Concerns, Department of Health, The City of New York; Associate Attending Physician, Department of Rheumatic Diseases, The Hospital for Joint Diseases, Beth Israel Medical Center; and Assistant Professor of Medicine, Mt. Sinai School of Medicine, City University of New York

Marshall Forstein, MD
Resident in Psychiatry, Massachusetts General Hospital; and Clinical Fellow in Psychiatry, Harvard Medical School

James P. Krajeski, MD
Private Practice of Psychiatry, San Francisco

Diego J. López, CSW
Clinical Director, Gay Men's Health Crisis, New York City; and Member, New York State AIDS Advisory Council

Carol C. Nadelson, MD
Professor of Psychiatry and Vice Chairman of Academic Affairs, Tufts University School of Medicine; and Director of Training and Education, Department of Psychiatry, New England Medical Center

Stuart E. Nichols, MD
Associate Chief, Medical and Psychiatric Services, Methadone Maintenance Treatment Program, Beth Israel Medical Center; and Senior Instructor in Psychiatry, Mt. Sinai School of Medicine, City University of New York

David G. Ostrow, MD, PhD

Associate Professor, Departments of Psychiatry and Community Health/ Preventive Medicine, Northwestern University School of Medicine; Director, Office of AIDS Activities, Chicago Department of Health; and Director of Research, Howard Brown Memorial Clinic

Harold Alan Pincus, MD

Special Assistant to the Director, National Institute of Mental Health

Michael W. Ross, BS Med, PhD

Senior Demonstrator in Psychiatry, South Australia Medical School, Flinders University

Rafael Tavares, MD

Director, Hispanic Psychiatric Clinic, Columbia Presbyterian Medical Center; and Instructor in Psychiatry, Columbia College of Physicians and Surgeons, Columbia University

Stanley R. Yancovitz, MD

Chief of Medicine and Drug Detoxification Service, Morris J. Berstein Institute, and Consultant in Infectious Disease, Beth Israel Medical Center; and Assistant Professor of Medicine, Mt. Sinai School of Medicine, City University of New York

Introduction

Acquired Immune Deficiency Syndrome (AIDS) has been declared "the public health threat of the century" (*Newsweek*, April 18, 1983), and the U.S. Surgeon General has designated it as the nation's number one health priority. Moralists have heightened public fear of the disease, and both God and "Nature" have been invoked in the debate. AIDS has been termed "Nature's revenge" against the "crime" of homosexuality. It has become like syphilis, leprosy, cancer, and bubonic plague, the contemporary metaphor for corruption, decay, and malignant, destructive, consummate evil.

The linking of AIDS with homosexual practice, minority populations, and others who are "alien" makes it susceptible to this metaphorical interpretation, as are other diseases that are transmitted through taboo behaviors (e.g., syphilis) or those with unknown etiologies (e.g., cancer). It is not clear whether AIDS is accidentally related to homosexuality or intrinsically so, and there is a danger of mistaken correlation with causality. A historic irony, the link between AIDS and syphilis, is found in the question of whether Columbus brought syphilis back to Europe in 1494 from Haiti(!) or whether it was caused by the mutation of an indigenous European organism (Charles Krauthammer, "The Politics of a Plague," *The New Republic*, August, 1983).

AIDS confronts us with a multitude of concerns about risk factors, susceptibility, contagion, and spread. Its priority as a health issue is not accidental, nor is it due to its prevalence. AIDS contains within it an intricate and complex dimension of the human condition; it encompasses the issues of individual values and social change. "Just as the gay community has been gaining tolerance, if not acceptance, AIDS has inflamed the most vicious homophobia —both among gays who cannot accept their own sexuality and among straights who consider the gay lifestyle a perverse crime against God, Nature, and all mankind" (*Boston Magazine*, February 1984).

Those studying AIDS experience both the desperation of victims and their families and the exciting promise of the scientific rewards that will ultimately be gained. In the exploration of this disease we may learn infinitely more about the human immune system and the multiconvergence of influences upon it than has previously been possible. Through research we may untangle many of the interrelationships between psychosocial factors and basic biologic processes, since this symptom complex may be caused by a familiar pathogen which has become more virulent in a highly susceptible group of patients. While we cannot be certain of susceptibility, it has been suggested that lifestyle, contact, and sexual practices are influential. Thus, fear, suspicion, hysteria, and even panic have emerged among many diverse groups.

The authors of this monograph have covered a vast expanse of information. They have clearly and succinctly described this disease as we now know it in order to replace myth and misunderstanding with information. This book may do much to change irrational societal anxiety.

In his chapter on epidemiology, Enlow emphasizes the importance and difficulty of obtaining accurate information when issues of confidentiality are most salient. Yancovitz's chapter on the medical aspects of AIDS is realistically pessimistic regarding the course of the illness, but he carefully and helpfully reviews the treatment interventions available for the successive complications which occur. Britton reminds clinicians that the disease may present with neurological symptoms easily (and incorrectly) viewed as psychiatric.

In the section of the book dedicated to the psychiatric treatment of AIDS, the authors describe what it is like to confront the unknown. In Forstein's chapter on AIDS anxiety, therapeutic approaches are proposed for those anxious about contracting AIDS so that they may gain a measure of control over their lives. Dilley, in his chapter on treatment issues, describes the pain of those who have already had a diagnosis made and thus must face an uncertain course. He emphasizes the illness as a continuum, "with certain common experiences and challenges to be mastered," and also suggests a number of approaches to facilitate coping. In the chapter on the psychiatric care of the seriously ill AIDS patient, Barbuto emphasizes the special characteristics of this group of patients who "suffer a dramatic change in self-esteem, daily habits, and general lifestyle in response to the illness." He also emphasizes the importance of considering organic mental syndromes that resemble functional psychiatric illness, and points to the need to recognize and treat the depressive symptoms that occur so frequently. Finally, Nichols emphasizes the importance of support networks for victims of AIDS who are usually isolated from friends and even family.

The authors of the section on social responses to AIDS consider the medical, psychological, and social issues presented by this catastrophic illness. Ostrow points out that the frustration, fear, and uncertainty that accompany epidemics of fatal diseases are clearly present with AIDS and lead to differences in the treatment that these patients receive. The isolation and stigmatization which AIDS victims experience call for us to examine our responses and make efforts to help them preserve their integrity and dignity. Tavares and López document the response of the gay community and applaud the support that has been offered by individuals and groups. Ross attempts to develop a psychological and social profile of AIDS, a "psychovenereology," so that some testable hypotheses may be generated. Pincus reinforces the need for research into the mental health aspects of AIDS and emphasizes the interrelationship between biologic and behavioral variables; further understanding of these conceptually separate factors can advance both psychiatry and medicine. Not only are studies necessary to delineate epidemiologic and risk factors with biobehavioral components, especially in the area of psychoimmunology and neuroendocrinology, but the behavioral and psychological consequences of AIDS for victims and their families and friends are enormous. As an epilogue, Krajeski presents a challenge to psychiatry and to society as a whole. He clarifies the role of psychiatry when confronted with AIDS-associated mental health problems and with the consequences of prejudice and stigmatization. He presses for preventive approaches as well as treatment.

The AIDS "epidemic" confronts us with our shared vulnerability, reinforced by myth, misperception, and fear. Control of this disease may force us to look more deeply at our values and attitudes, and it may necessitate changes in lifestyles, public health programs, and research. Our humanity, however, must guide us toward care and love, as first priorities.

Carol C. Nadelson, M.D.
President-Elect
American Psychiatric Association

MEDICAL ASPECTS

This section is designed to give practicing psychiatrists an overview of the epidemiologic, immunologic, medical, and neurological conditions encountered with AIDS. The information contained herein should facilitate the understanding of some of the problems encountered in these disciplines and assist therapists in coordinating the care of their patients. Of special note are the discussions of the difficulties involved in making a diagnosis of AIDS; the impossibility, at this time, of separating the prodromal syndrome of AIDS from nonspecific conditions; the misuse of protective measures that are both counterproductive and dehumanizing; and the numerous neurologic problems that resemble and sometimes present as psychiatric illness. All persons working with AIDS must be aware that the disease has not spread to the general population to any great degree and that the percentage of cases in each of the affected subgroups of our society has remained remarkably constant. Therefore, it is apparent—despite frightening reports that continue to appear in the news media—that AIDS is difficult to transmit from person to person and cannot be spread by casual contact.

1

Epidemiology and Immunology of Acquired Immune Deficiency Syndrome

Roger W. Enlow, M.D.

1

Epidemiology and Immunology of Acquired Immune Deficiency Syndrome

It was recognized in the spring of 1981 that two unusual and seemingly dissimilar outbreaks of Kaposi's sarcoma (KS) and *Pneumocystis carinii* pneumonia (PCP) were occurring in gay men and intravenous drug users. These outbreaks were discovered by piecing together case reports from Los Angeles and New York with the requests made to the Centers for Disease Control (CDC) for the drug pentamidine, used exclusively to treat PCP. Ongoing surveillance of outbreaks at federal, state, and local levels soon led to the inclusion of other opportunistic infections. The discovery of an underlying immune defect in all of these conditions prompted the adoption of the name acquired immune deficiency syndrome (AIDS) in the late summer of 1981, despite some reluctance because of uncertainty about etiology and possible confusion with known abnormal immune conditions which occur in various diseases.

EPIDEMIOLOGY

For the purposes of this chapter, it may be helpful to differentiate between the terms "surveillance" and "epidemiology." Surveillance is the broad overview of a disease process which begins to elucidate its patterns; it is a kind of rough, but accurate epidemiology. Epidemiology involves investigation of a disease in depth, beginning with surveillance data, to delineate its full natural history and to characterize its etiology. Most data now available for AIDS are surveillance rather than epidemiological in character.

For the purpose of collecting comparable data throughout the United States, the CDC narrowly defined a reportable case of AIDS as the occurrence of a reliably diagnosed disease at least moderately indicative of a defect in cell-mediated immunity in the absence of a known or identifiable underlying cause for that defect. Specifically excluded are the immune deficiencies associated with myelo- and lymphoproliferative diseases (such as leukemias and lymphomas), autoimmune disorders (like systemic lupus erythematosus and rheumatoid arthritis), and the corticosteroid, cytotoxic, or radiation therapy for these and other illnesses. Cases of KS in persons over 60 years of age were also excluded because they might represent the known but rare form of that neoplasm. Hypogammaglobulinemia and congenital immune deficiencies are also excluded from the CDC case definition of AIDS.

The restrictive CDC case definition does not necessarily represent the full spectrum of AIDS, but the case definition is necessary to ensure uniformity in prospective reporting by physicians to public health agencies. A fuller definition of the disorders must await data from the more detailed epidemiologic studies and the basic research that is now being conducted by many health care institutions throughout the world.

The prodromal syndrome for AIDS has not been fully elucidated. Conditions such as persistent, generalized lymphadenopathy, idiopathic thrombocytopenia, leukopenia, and reactivated varicella-zoster virus infections have been seen in some persons who later developed AIDS. However, others with these conditions have not developed it, and the use of terms like "pre-AIDS," "lesser AIDS," "prodromal AIDS," or "AIDS related complex" (ARC) is probably premature, scientifically confusing, and potentially stigmatizing to persons with these nonspecific conditions. Hopefully, the long-term prospective studies now underway, together with basic science breakthroughs, will define the AIDS precursor state more clearly.

Based on the early observation that AIDS was occurring in several specific groups, it was assumed that other individuals in these groups were at increased risk for acquiring the disease or for being exposed to it. The CDC and other agencies began assigning each case to groups according to presumed risk factors or social group. The initial groups used in the CDC classification were homosexual males, intravenous drug abusers, and a scattering of others who did not fit into the first two categories. To avoid double counting, a single case could only be listed in one group. Thus a gay man who used intravenous drugs was only assigned to the "homosexual male" group. Some of the serious limitations to this system came to light when bisexual men were found to have AIDS. The decision as to which category an individual case belonged was based on the impression of the reporting physician. Given the difficulties of obtaining information regarding confidential, perhaps embarrassing (to patient or physician), and sometimes illicit activities, and considering the circumstances of the interview, the reliability of the CDC's tabulations must be suspect. Despite these problems, this mutually exclusive system persists to the present in most reports. The group of individuals with more than one risk factor is now about 8 percent of the national case total, which may in fact be an underestimate.

Further problems developed when cases of AIDS among Haitians and hemophiliacs and suspected transfusion-related cases were reported. It remains unclear as to why Haitians (in the United States and Haiti) have AIDS despite considerable, and often damaging, speculations. It is certainly not clear that they developed AIDS as a result of the fact that they were born and lived in Haiti, but the creation of a separate risk group for Haitians gives undue credence to a causal implication. This has prompted a review of the entire system of risk groups with some early changes in the reporting of surveillance data from the New York City Department of Health.

The problems of classification remain for the time being. Medical, scientific, and public attention has been focused on the comparatively few hemophiliac and transfusion-related cases. The possibility that the nation's blood supply was contaminated with a factor or factors that might induce AIDS precipitated a series of intense discussions and hasty ill-advised actions in some cases. The implication of blood and blood products as a cause of AIDS in some cases is still under careful evaluation. The entire epidemiologic pattern of AIDS is similar to that of other blood-borne infections, including hepatitis B and non-A, non-B hepatitis. It is interesting to note that the latter disease, as with AIDS, does not have a specific blood marker to identify carriers who are potentially hazardous blood donors. The recognition and natural history of both diseases is thus completely based on epidemiologic or surveillance data at this time.

Since the outset of AIDS surveillance, there have been a small and interesting number of individuals without identified "risk factors." Some of these persons died before an adequate interview could be obtained. Some may involve cases of KS or the other opportunistic processes that are not related to the current AIDS epidemic, while a few of these persons have been sexual partners of intravenous drug users or gay men and not themselves members of a "risk group." Still other persons with AIDS may simply not have responded accurately to the questions asked about private, sensitive aspects of their lives. A number of factors influence case-reporting patterns in any given month. These factors include public awareness of the disease; reporting requirements by city, state, and other public health authorities; and the degree to which case finding is an active or passive process. During the early months of 1983, the New York City Department of Health, in cooperation with the CDC, piloted hospital surveillance of AIDS through infection control officers and clinical investigators involved in the care of inpatients with AIDS. Specially trained public health advisors were enlisted to visit hospitals and assist in the process of reporting newly identified cases while clarifying information about those already reported. This resulted in a transient rise in the number of cases reported, but there was no change in the number of cases when they were listed by the date of diagnosis. Because the time between diagnosis and reporting may vary considerably, the number of new cases reported in any given month does not accurately reflect the true number diagnosed in that period. This has recently resulted in the misperception that the number of newly diagnosed cases is diminishing when, in fact, the numbers continue to increase over time, although not necessarily at the rapid rate of late 1982.

Concerns about confidentiality of an individual's personal and medical information similarly contribute to variation in the month-to-month reporting of cases. Considerable improvement in awareness about this issue and, in some cases, improvement in the actual level of protection provided to patients has contributed to better reporting patterns. Modification of a local health code, such as protecting the records from subpoena, is a step in the right direction. More statutory protection of patient confidentiality is clearly needed.

Our present understanding of the pattern of disease varies tremendously from one risk group to another, as does the presenting problem which brings the person with AIDS to medical attention. Persons with a history of intravenous drug use are more likely to present with an opportunistic infection, while gay men are more likely to have KS as their initial manifestation. Mortality is greater in persons with opportunistic infections than in those with KS. The overall reported mortality has been placed at 40 percent but has increased over time for those persons diagnosed early in the epidemic. The true mortality and natural history of this disease will not be known for some time. Significant differences in the racial and ethnic mix of these groups and, hence, the secondary associations between race and the disease process have been noted. There has been considerable recent attention to the possibility that genetic factors, such as the human leukocyte antigen (HLA) system or related cell-surface determinants, might be in some way contributory to a particular complication or outcome of the syndrome. Although, to date, there has been no confirmed report of recovery from AIDS, the possibility may exist.

When the rate of increase of AIDS for each of the major risk groups is put in graph form, the resultant curves are similar, despite the differences in course and mortality. Even the numerically smaller groups, such as hemophiliacs and pediatric cases, produce curves with slopes of increase which resemble the major groups. Of importance, when comparing the latter two groups with the others, is the apparent absence of identifiable AIDS-related problems prior to late 1978. This has led to the conclusion, supported by retrospective surveys of pneumonia deaths in intravenous drug users and hemophiliacs and reviews of medical records and pathological reports on lymphadenopathy, that AIDS is a new phenomenon in the United States.

Attempts to understand these curves and to construct mathematical models of them is made difficult by the compounding variables mentioned above. In New York City, for the third quarter of 1983, there was a slight and perhaps significant decrease in the rate of increase in AIDS. Caution is essential in interpreting this change, however, and continued reassessment, over time, will be needed before it is clear that such a trend exists.

Internationally, 267 cases of AIDS, in 21 countries, were listed by the World Health Organization in November 1983. The epidemiological trends in these cases are less clear than in the United States, which may be due, in part, to a delay in the recognition of the syndrome. Efforts to clarify this picture are now underway. The epidemiologic curve of new cases for each of these countries is, again, similar to that for AIDS reported in the United States. Suggestions made about the origin of AIDS have been premature and damaging to the groups affected and the work in progress designed to shed light on the question.

Since surveillance began, one of the essential concerns has been to detect spread beyond the apparent sociologic and geographic categories outlined. The occurrence of AIDS in hemophiliacs and blood recipients increased the concern still further. The reports of children with AIDS or AIDS-like illnesses raised the possibility of household spread, albeit to perhaps a particularly vulnerable population. Despite these concerns, when the affected groups are reviewed over the entire time of the epidemic, the percentages of cases in each category have remained nearly constant. Moreover, despite awareness that occupational exposure of health-care workers probably preceded actual diagnosis of the disease, there are only a few reports of AIDS in health-care workers who do not have a known risk factor. Even these few cases, when carefully reviewed, fail to show a causal relationship of exposure to patients with AIDS. The best infection control guidelines are those already established for blood-borne infections in general. Specific "AIDS precautions" are unwarranted and can stigmatize patients and produce confusion, which may even reduce caution in the laboratory and at the bedside. Often the unmarked tube of blood in the lab is more hazardous than the specifically labelled one.

IMMUNOLOGY

The immunologic abnormalities associated with AIDS are complicated and inadequately understood at this time. Since the earliest reported cases, there have been persistent hematologic findings including leukopenia (most frequently a lymphopenia), occasional anemia, and thrombocytopenia. Atypical lymphocytes with monocytoid characteristics are also seen. These observations, together with the types of opportunistic infections that patients developed, prompted further investigations of the lymphopenia using immunofluorescent monoclonal antibodies.

Monclonal antibodies are a new research tool which have helped to define the structure and function of the immune system in recent years. They allow the research scientist to detect specific subsets of lymphocytes which have particular functions within the immune system, such as the T-helper (also known as T-inducer or T_4) cells and the T-suppressor (also knows as T_8) cells. T cells are identified by specific antigens on the surface of the cells (the "cell surface markers"). Monoclonal antibodies are attracted to these antigens, and when the antibodies are made fluorescent, the various types of T cells can be seen and counted using special microscopes. This delicate and laborious technique has led to the discovery that AIDS patients have an abnormality in the ratio of T-helper to T-suppressor cells (the H/S ratio), which, in AIDS, is caused by a reduction in the number of helper cells in the peripheral blood. In a healthy state there are about twice as many helper as there are suppressor cells.

The measurement of the subsets of T cells is principally used in immunology research; many technical problems make it difficult to perform and interpret. In definite cases of AIDS, however, the finding of decreased helper cells is consistent. Abnormalities in H/S ratios and a decrease in helper cells are sometimes found among healthy persons from an AIDS "risk group" or even in gay men with persistent lymphadenopathy or other nonspecific conditions. The significance of these findings, however, is not yet understood but is being carefully evaluated in prospective studies. T-cell counts are useful primarily in confirming a clinical picture or in following subjects in a research protocol, but they are not a screening test for AIDS.

Table 1 summarizes the known laboratory abnormalities in AIDS. The detectable circulating interferon may be an abnormal form of this substance. Alpha-1-thymosin acts to stimulate T cells. In addition, it has been reported that the number and function of natural killer cells (some of which are probably another subset of T cells) is diminished, that there is a decreased and delayed lymphocyte proliferation in response to mitogens, and that T helper cells function inadequately even when sufficient in number. Finally, despite antibody titers which suggest immunity to a specific virus, there may be a deficiency in the cytolytic and cytotoxic capacity of the immune system to that virus in patients with AIDS.

Full understanding of these findings is impossible at this time; they involve the perplexing research frontiers in immunology. It is clear, however, that in AIDS there is a defect in the cellular component of the immune system. T cells are thymus-dependent lymphocytes (the cell-mediated branch of the immune system) as contrasted to the B cells, which are bone marrow–dependent lymphocytes (the humoral branch of the immune system, the B cells producing antibodies). Cellular immunity is important in resolving acute viral infections and in preventing the recrudescence of latent viruses, and its mechanism of action in this context is now the subject of many research efforts. The role of cell surface markers other than those which are associated with helper or suppressor functions is also being explored, particularly those known to be part of the self-recognition function of the immune system (such as HLA markers). Determining which of these abnormalities are primary to AIDS, and which are secondary to the opportunistic infections, will take some time to sort out.

Serologic tests may be invalid in AIDS. T-helper cells induce B cells to produce antibodies; therefore, with decreased T-helper cells the results of serologic testing may be difficult to interpret. In addition, the reactivation of an old illness which can occur in AIDS would stimulate the B cells to produce increased levels of antibodies. For example, reactivation of mononucleosis would

Table 1 Typical Laboratory Abnormalities in Patients with AIDS

Parameter	Abnormality
Hemoglobin and Hematocrit	Normal or slightly decreased
Routine White Blood Cell Count	Normal or decreased
WBC Differential Counts	
Lymphocytes	Normal, increased, or decreased (if increased, often with atypical lymphocytes; if decreased, the T helper cells are markedly reduced)
Monocytes	Normal to increased with atypical lymphocytes frequently mistaken for monocytes
T Lymphocyte Subsets (defined by monoclonal antibodies)	
Total T helper lymphocytes	Decreased (usually less than 500/mm^3 of whole blood)
Total T suppressor lymphocytes	Normal or slightly increased (usually 500–800/mm^3 of whole blood)
Helper/Suppressor T Cell Ratio*	Decreased, persistently less than 1.0
Lymphocyte Stimulation Responses to mitogens such as phytohemagglutinin A, concanavalin A, and pokeweed mitogen antigen	Decreased thymidine uptake
Platelet Counts	Normal or decreased due to antibodies which may be part of immune complexes on their surface
Natural Killer Cell Activity	Decreased
Virus-Specific Cytotoxic Activity	Decreased
Quantitative Immunoglobulins	Normal or increased
Circulating Immune Complexes	Present by C1q binding, Raji cells, and other assays

NOTE. Other serologic abnormalities in AIDS: circulating acid-labile (alpha) interferon may be present and similar to that seen in certain autoimmune diseases; elevated levels of alpha-1-thymosin, a T lymphocyte stimulator; and elevated levels of beta-2-microglobulin, a low-molecular-weight protein associated with the class I histocompatibility antigens suggesting a high turn-over rate of cells or cell-surface structures.

* A low helper/suppressor T cell ratio is not indicative of AIDS when it is caused by an increase in T-suppressor cells (which commonly occurs in viral and other infections). In AIDS the low ratio is the result of a reduction in T-helper cells.

result in increased circulating antibodies to Epstein-Barr virus. Because these standard diagnostic tools may be unreliable, invasive procedures which facilitate a histologic or culture diagnosis are often essential in the evaluation of an AIDS patient. Thus, a tissue biopsy might be called for in a patient with central nervous system disease or pneumonia when, normally, serologic titers might be diagnostic.

The production of immune complexes and their clearance is part of the healthy response of the body to foreign proteins, other substances, and infections. In AIDS, the evaluation of the circulating immune complexes is even more unclear than the monoclonal antibody studies. Several different techniques are commonly used to measure them with significant differences in what they recognize. Most rely on the presence of an antibody molecule attached to an antigen. The nature of the circulating immune complexes is being intensively studied and may in time lead to important insights into the cause of AIDS.

One of the oldest methods of assessing immune function is skin testing to elicit an anamnestic or recalled response. Skin tests measure delayed-type hypersensitivity, an indication of cellular immunity. However, the variability in the antigens used and in the methods of applying them has contributed to uncertainty about their role in AIDS. The standard intradermal application has been used in many of the studies reporting to date. Some of these studies have observed anergy, but careful efforts to induce sensitization suggest that an impaired response is more characteristic of AIDS. The recent introduction of standardized antigens and application systems that are reproducible, such as Multitest by l'Institut Mérieux, have great promise as clinical tools for prospective studies.

Commercially available "AIDS screening tests" often purport to offer the clinician a useful battery of tests as a package with a bargain price tag. However, in light of the complicated immunologic abnormalities of the syndrome, the value of these determinations and their potential for harm must be carefully considered. It is best to proceed cautiously and in consultation with experienced investigators when ordering and interpreting these tests, so as to avoid costly mistakes and misinformation which may result when research tools are used prematurely for clinical care.

ETIOLOGY: THE ROLE OF HTLV III

On April 23, 1984, Margaret Heckler, Secretary of Health and Human Services, announced that a probable cause of AIDS had been found. Dr. Robert Gallo and others at the National Cancer Institute had isolated and characterized a new human T lymphotrophic virus that was preliminarily designated as HTLV III.

Dr. Gallo's findings opened several new horizons. He also reported an improved method for growing and recovering HTLV III, one that utilizes a special host cell derived from the human T cell and that is similar to normal T helper (or T_4) lymphocytes. The cell that hosts the virus grows well under laboratory conditions without itself being destroyed by the viral replication and release into the surrounding culture medium. The virus can be seen budding from the surface of the host cell and can be recultured in fresh hosts. This provides the large quantities of virus necessary to perform detailed studies of its structure and behavior. Importantly, it has already led to the development of research techniques to detect it.

Dr. Gallo has been working for many years on factors that make lymphocytes grow. He previously identified the T cell growth factor (TCGF), which is now known as interleukin 2. He also isolated the original human T cell virus, HTLV I. The initials HTLV then stood for human T cell leukemia virus, after the type of leukemia from which it was first obtained. HTLV I is quite peculiar in that its genetic material is of one type, RNA, and it contains a protein or enzyme called reverse transcriptase, which is capable of making a DNA copy of an RNA substance. This method of copying is the opposite of all known systems for transcribing genes, and its discovery has led, in part, to the genetic engineering revolution.

HTLV I enters its target cell, a T lymphocyte, and makes DNA copies of its RNA genetic code, thereby altering the T cell's genetic code. Some of this material is passed along through the next cycle of cell growth and division; this is thought to be an important model which may explain the role of the viruses in certain kinds of cancer and disease. Although rare, T cell leukemia exists worldwide. A concentration of cases, however, has been found in several generations of certain families in Southern Japan, which may indicate that HTLV I can be passed from parent to offspring during conception.

In 1983 both Harvard University and the CDC reported finding weak reactions to HTLV I in the blood of some persons with AIDS. The reaction was not found often or strongly enough to make HTLV I a leading contender as the cause of AIDS, but it did suggest that an organism related to it might be involved.

Early reports in the Spring of 1983 from l'Institut Pasteur suggested that a retrovirus, the lymphadenopathy associated virus (LAV), was associated with AIDS. LAV should soon be fully characterized and compared to HTLV III. Many scientists feel that it should grow as well as HTLV III in the new host cell, and in fact may be the same virus. It is of considerable importance to compare these viruses and other isolates obtained from AIDS patients from different parts of the world. If they are shown to be alike and are not found in persons who do not have or develop AIDS, these results would strongly support the idea that they are the cause of AIDS.

HTLV III has been isolated from 48 different specimens. It has been found in persons with AIDS and in persons with what has been termed pre-AIDS or AIDS related complex (ARC). It has also been recovered from three of four healthy mothers of children with AIDS, and one of 22 healthy gay men. The one healthy gay man from whom HTLV III was cultured has subsequently developed AIDS, in contrast to all the mothers tested who remain healthy at this time. This result suggests that other factors may play a role in producing the disease in exposed hosts. Using the large quantities of virus now available; Dr. Gallo's research group has shown that HTLV III is similar to, but different from, the other known members of the HTLV family. In addition to the presence of reverse transcriptase, they all seem to have a specificity for T_4 cells. Unlike the new culture method, HTLV III injures and destroys T-helper cells by mechanisms which are at the moment unclear. In the human body this could result in the eventual reduction in the absolute number of T_4 cells, a finding peculiar to AIDS. HTLV III may also impair T-helper cells in other ways. Interleukin 2 is essential for T cell growth and maturation, and, so far as is known, it is only produced by T_4 cells. It is possible that the loss of only a few, critical, interleukin 2–producing T_4 cells might seriously compromise the ability of this cell line to replenish itself.

Besides the isolation of HTLV III, Dr. Gallo also reported the ability to detect antibodies to this virus in blood samples. Of the blood tested to date, positive HTLV III reactions were found in 88 percent of persons with AIDS and 79 percent of persons with symptoms suggesting ARC, but in less than 1 percent of the blood donor population. As with other conditions, the presence of antibodies may be an indication of exposure rather than active disease. It is not known if these antibodies are protective once the disease has been established, and other major questions still need to be answered before the presence of antibodies to HTLV III can be properly interpreted and of clinical use.

An example of some of the problems involved may be illustrated by the problem of testing for hepatitis B, where the presence of one type of antibody indicates exposure, another implies protection, and still other tests looking for viral structure indicate the actual presence of the virus. Furthermore, these tests do not all have the same significance in determining who is infectious and who is not. Intensive efforts are now underway to develop an understanding of similar concepts in AIDS.

Development of a safe, effective vaccine and improved therapeutic measures for those already suffering with AIDS are not likely to be seen in the near future, but they will undoubtedly be found much sooner because of the scientific breakthroughs of the National Cancer Institute and l'Institut Pasteur.

2

Medical Aspects of Acquired Immune Deficiency Syndrome

Stanley R. Yancovitz, M.D.

2

Medical Aspects of Acquired Immune Deficiency Syndrome

Acquired immune deficiency syndrome (AIDS) is defined by the occurrence of infections and neoplasms which indicate a severe abnormality of the patients' immune system, particularly the cell-mediated arm, without a known underlying cause such as lymphoma or long-term immunosuppressive or corticosteroid therapy (1). The patient may present with an infection such as *Pneumocystic carinii* pneumonia (PCP) or disseminated Kaposi's sarcoma (KS) which confirms the diagnosis of AIDS. Table 1 presents the current list of infections generally thought to substantiate a clinical diagnosis of AIDS. Other patients present with a subacute or chronic syndrome of malaise, fatigue, low-grade fever, nonspecific diarrhea, or puzzling neuromuscular or rheumatological complaints. Without a reliable diagnostic test, and in view of the dire implications of the diagnosis, most clinicians are loath to make a diagnosis of "AIDS prodrome" or "pre-AIDS" in these patients. Thorough investigations for a variety of disorders that can cause similar symptoms, signs, and laboratory abnormalities and follow-up with long-term prospective studies are necessary to determine the ultimate outcome of this diverse group. Depending on the findings in each case, a diligent search should be made for syphilis, hepatitis, lymphadenopathic toxoplasmosis, disseminated mycobacterial and fungal diseases, endocarditis, infectious diarrhea, lymphoma, and collagen vascular disease.

The clinical work-up of these patients should include a complete blood count, differential leukocyte count, platelet count, chest roentgenogram, urinalysis, blood chemistries, and tuberculin skin testing with purified protein derivative and control antigens. A thorough imminological work-up should also be done. Any suspicious symptoms or pulmonary findings detected by radiology should be evaluated carefully. Gallium scanning has been helpful in screening for active pulmonary infections in AIDS patients with normal or equivocal chest roentgenograms (author's unpublished observation). Pneumonic processes commonly require invasive diagnostic procedures. Diffuse pulmonary processes are generally approached by bronchoscopy with histologic and cytologic studies using special stains and cultures for bacteria, mycobacteria, viruses, *Pneumocystis*, *Legionella*, and fungi. Open-lung biopsy is used in some centers, but most clinicians use it only when bronchoscopy is nondiagnostic or not feasible.

Lymph node biopsy may diagnose disseminated mycobacterial and fungal infections, lymphomas, and KS (which may appear only in the lymph nodes). Additionally, some centers have

Table 1 Infectious Diseases Characteristic of AIDS Patients That Are Probably Diagnostic in Absence of a Known Cause of Immunosuppression

Any of the following:
Pneumocystis carinii pneumonia
Disseminated infection due to cytomegalovirus or herpes simplex virus
Locally destructive and persistent lesions due to herpes simplex virus (duration of over five weeks)
Disseminated nontuberculous mycobacterial infection
Chronic diarrhea due to *Cryptosporidium* (duration of over two months)
Disseminated or cerebral infection due to *Toxoplasma* (in an adult)
Disseminated cryptococcal infection
Multifocal leukoencephalopathy

Also suspicious:
Disseminated tuberculosis
Severe oral moniliasis or esophageal moniliasis
Desseminated varicella-zoster virus infection
Recurrent salmonella and shigella bacteremias
Infections caused by organisms whose major defense mechanism is cell-mediated immunity not yet clearly associated with increased incidence or severity in AIDS patients

reported serial nonspecific histologic changes in lymph nodes which seem to correlate with disease progression (2). Unless there is a specific investigational protocol, lymph node biopsy in the individual patient should be performed only when it is likely to answer a specific clinical question (such as whether lymphoma or disseminated infection is present or why a sudden change in size or characteristics of the lymph node has occurred) or to evaluate a febrile illness or significant deterioration.

Special stains for acid-fast bacilli (AFB) and fungi are indicated in all biopsies, even in the absence of granulomas or other histological abnormalities. Bone marrow biopsy and culture is helpful in diagnosing disseminated mycobacterial and fungal infection. Special blood culture techniques may reveal mycobacteria (3).

Patients with diarrhea should have stools examined for bacteria, ova, and parasites. Special stains should be done to identify cryptosporidia and masses of atypical mycobacteria.

The invasiveness and expense of many of the above procedures mandates the use of good clinical judgment in the evaluation of these patients. A thorough baseline evaluation and clinical follow-up are necessary.

Initial and serial serologic studies for toxoplasmosis and cytomegalovirus (CMV) may be of use in interpreting subsequent clinical events. Banked sera may be helpful in the future when a specific diagnostic test becomes available, especially now that the probable cause of AIDS has been isolated. It is unclear whether treating for occult, asymptomatic, or possibly symptomatic lymph node toxoplasmosis is indicated; however, since patients can present with necrotizing toxoplasma encephalitis as their first manifestation of AIDS, some centers favor testing and prophylactic treatment. On the other hand, AIDS patients have an exceedingly high incidence of reactions to the sulfa drugs required to treat toxoplasmosis. Similarly, the impetus to prescribe prophylactic treatment for PCP with trimethoprim-sulfamethoxazole is tempered by the likelihood of hypersensitive or toxic reactions (4).

The administration of pneumococcal and influenza vaccines may be worthwhile early in the course of the illness. There is evidence that, in the late stages of other illnesses characterized by severe deficits in cell-mediated immunity, the ability to respond to these vaccines with appropriate levels of humoral antibodies diminishes as the disease progresses (5).

The retrospective study of AIDS patients shows that, in addition to variable degrees of diffuse lymphadenopathy, the prodromal syndrome may include retinal exudates and either new or more extensive common skin ailments, such as seborrheic dermatitis. The development of extensive oral thrush, retinal lesions consistent with CMV retinitis (hemorrhages and exudates that tend to streak along the retinal vessels), persistent oral or genital herpes (greater than three weeks), or disseminated herpes zoster seems to be particularly ominous in the course of the prodromal syndrome.

Any suspicious skin lesions appearing in persons at risk for AIDS should be biopsied to rule out KS. If KS is diagnosed at one site, patients require endoscopic evaluation for disseminated disease in the gastrointestinal tract. They should also have dermatologic consultation to detect other skin lesions. Several chemotherapeutic regimens, including vincristine and its derivatives, combination chemotherapy, interferon, and radiation, all may cause KS lesions to shrink or disappear. These various treatment regimens remain in experimental stages since it is yet to be shown that they enhance survival in these patients. Patients with disseminated KS involving visceral organs seem to have a poor prognosis despite therapy. The enhanced susceptibility to opportunistic infections that may ensue from immunosuppressive therapies must be kept in mind. In addition, some patients with KS appear to follow a relatively benign clinical course, similar to the classic form of the disease.

Candidal mucosal infections can be treated with topical nystatin, oral ketaconazole, or parenteral amphotericin B for severe and persistent lesions. There seems to be an increased risk of side effects to ketaconazole with AIDS patients. Herpes simplex and zoster frequently respond to antiviral agents such as acyclovir and vidarabine. However, herpes simplex virus infections commonly recur, and despite antiviral therapy, they may become resistant and cause progressively destructive local and systemic disease. CMV may cause progressive retinitis and blindness, central ner-

Table 2 Pathogens Involved in Clinical Syndromes Produced in AIDS Patients

Infectious Organism	Manifestations	Diagnosis	Treatment
Viruses			
Herpes simplex virus	Destructive vesicular and ulcerative lesions in oral and genital area, disseminated infection, retinitis	Tzank prep, viral culture	Vidarabine, acyclovir
Varicella-zoster virus	Zoster, disseminated zoster	Appearance, viral culture, cytology, Tzank prep	Vidarabine, acyclovir
Cytomegalovirus	Retinitis, encephalitis, pneumonia, adrenal necrosis, enterocolitis	Histology, viral culture, ?serology not diagnostic, CT scans	None available
Adenovirus	?Significant in AIDS	Viral culture (oral, eye)	None available
Papovavirus	Progressive multifocal leukoencephalopathy	Biopsy, ?electron microscopy	Vidarabine
Epstein-Barr virus	?Role in etiology ?Cause of polyclonal gammopathy	Viral culture, serology	None available
Retroviruses			
Human T cell lymphotrophic virus type, III (HTLV III)	Probable role in etiology	Special culture, serology	None available
Lymphadenopathy-associated virus (LAV)	Probable role in etiology	Special culture, serology	None available
Bacteria			
Legionella pneumophila	Pneumonia, encephalopathy, renal insufficiency	Culture (special media), direct fluorescent stain of sputum, transtracheal aspiration, bronchoscopy or biopsy specimen, serology (in AIDS)	Erythromycin and/or rifampin

Mycobacterium tuberculosis, nontuberculous mycobacteria	Pulmonary or disseminated disease	Sputum, bronchoscopy	Isoniazid, rifampin, others
Mycobacterium avium-intracellulare	Pulmonary or disseminated disease	Lumbar puncture (special technique; blood culture), lymph node biopsy, liver biopsy, bone marrow biopsy	?Ansamycin, clofazimine, multiple antituberculosis medications
Salmonella	Enterocolitis	Culture	Ampicillin
Shigella	Recurrent bacteremia	Culture	Trimethoprim-sulfamethoxazole, chloramphenicol (depends on sensitivity)
Fungi			
Candida	Oral, esophageal, disseminated	Appearance, smear, culture, biopsy	Nystatin, ketaconazole, amphotericin B, 5-flucytosine
Cryptococcus	Pulmonary, central nervous system	India ink staining, culture, cryptococcal antigen in blood, CSF, and urine, biopsy	Amphotericin B, 5-flucytosine, ?ketaconazole
Parasites			
Pneumocystis carinii	Pneumonia, ?eye, ?brain, ?bone marrow	Biopsy, bronchoscopy, or open cytology	Trimethoprim-sulfamethoxazole, pentamidine
Toxoplasma	Encephalitis, pneumonia, lymphadenopathy, retinitis	?Serology, biopsy, animal inoculation	Sulfadiazine, pyramethamine, ?clindamycin, ?spiramycin
Cryptosporidium	Enterocolitis, ?dissemination	Stool examination (special technique), stain for acid-fast bacilli, Shearers modified methylene blue	None available
Isospora belli	Diarrhea	Stool examination	Trimethoprim-sulfamethoxazole
Strongyloides stercoralis	Diarrhea, hyperinfestation syndrome, disseminated disease, second-degree bacteremias	Larvae seen on examination of stool, duodenal fluid, or other secretions	Thiabendazole

vous system disease (which is discussed in Chapter 3), pneumonia, and multisystem destructive changes involving the liver, spleen, bowel, and adrenal glands. There is no effective treatment currently available for CMV infections.

Pneumonia in an AIDS patient may be due to an expanding list of pathogens. These include the routine causes of pneumonia, such as *Pneumococcus* and *Mycoplasma*, as well as *Legionella*, *Pneumocystis*, *Mycobacterium tuberculosis*, nontuberculous mycobacteria, *Cryptococcus*, CMV, and *Toxoplasma*. Combined infection with two or more of these pathogens is common. Almost all of these agents can cause disseminated disease.

Patients with AIDS and those with the prodromal syndrome may demonstrate a variety of hematological abnormalities, including the anemia of chronic disease with high serum ferritin values, neutropenia, lymphocytopenia, and thrombocytopenia. The thrombocytopenia has been associated with high platelet-associated IgG and C3 in some patients (6). The role of viruses (such as CMV) or the putative AIDS agent in the production of these cytopenias remains to be investigated. Corticosteroid therapy and splenectomy have been used successfully to treat severe thrombocytopenia, but decisions to employ these measures have to be carefully considered. Many patients seem to tolerate very low platelet counts for an extended period of time without major hemorrhage, perhaps because the platelets are young and enzyme-rich when a peripheral destructive (splenic) process is present.

Fever may be caused by an extensive list of conditions, and it demands a careful and systematic approach with the judicious use of serological testing, radiology, computerized tomography scans, lumbar punctures, nuclear scans, routine and special culture techniques, invasive surgical procedures, and occasional clinical trials. It is important not to overlook common causes of fever, especially in debilitated AIDS patients, for they are clearly at risk for nosocomial infections such as catheter sepsis and aspiration pneumonia.

Table 2 lists the pathogens by each type of infectious agent (viruses, bacteria, fungi, and parasites), the clinical syndromes each can produce in AIDS patients, and the diagnostic techniques and treatment for each that are currently available. It is anticipated that this list will expand both in number of pathogens and the extent of pathophysiological alterations attributed to them.

High levels of circulating immune complexes and polyclonal immunoglobulin elevation are present in many patients. The relationship of these findings to the unexplained rheumatologic, neurologic, and hematologic abnormalities in some patients needs further investigation.

Patient comfort and adequate nursing care, especially in debilitated or terminally ill patients, assumes priority in treatment decisions. Published guidelines of the preventive measures to be used in the hospital setting offer several alternatives (7, 8). It is most important that the infection control office coordinate sensible measures in a uniform manner that will allow for maximum patient care and safety and minimum risk or anxiety for staff and visitors.

The diagnosis, by current definitions, cannot be made in patients who have an underlying cause of immunosuppression, but who are also in a risk group for AIDS. An example of such a patient is found in a bisexual man who had been medicating himself with high doses of prednisone for what may have been prodromal symptoms. He presented with PCP and subsequently died of cryptococcal meningitis. It would seem wise to apply the AIDS prevention measures with these patients.

Thus far, the AIDS patient who is cured of one complication is left at risk for recurrence, or serial and combined complications, because of the persistent and irreversible state of immunosuppression.

In summary, the clinician must guide the patient through a maze of diagnostic and therapeutic options. He or she must deal with the present uncertainties of diagnosis in the possible prodromal patients—and deal with the successive complications and the dire prognosis of the full AIDS syndrome.

References

1. Centers for Disease Control: Pneumocystitis pneumonia, Los Angeles. MMWR 30:250–252, 1981

2. Fernandez R, Mouradian J, Metroka C, et al: The prognostic value of histopathology in persistent generalized lymphadenopathy in homosexual men. N Engl J Med 309:185–186, 1983

3. Macher A, Kovacs J, Gill V, et al: Bacteremia due to *Mycobacterium avium-intracellulare* in the acquired immunodeficiency syndrome. Ann Intern Med 99:782–785, 1983

4. Jaffe NS, Abrams DI, Amman A, et al: Complications of cotrimoxazole in treatment of AIDS-associated *Pneumocystis* pneumonia in homosexual men. Lancet 2:1109–1111, 1983

5. Weitzman S, Aisenberg A, Siber G, et al: Impaired humoral immunity in treated Hodgkins disease. N Engl J Med 297:245–248, 1977

6. Morvis L, Distengeld A, Amorosi E, et al: Autoimmune thrombocytopenic purpura in homosexual men. Ann Intern Med 96:714–717, 1982

7. Centers for Disease Control: Acquired Immune Deficiency Syndrome (AIDS): Precautions for clinical and laboratory staffs. MMWR 31:577–580, 1982

8. Conte J, Hadley W, Sande M: Infection control guidelines for patients with the acquired immune deficiency syndrome (AIDS). N Engl J Med 309:740–744, 1983

3

Neurology of Acquired Immune Deficiency Syndrome

Carolyn B. Britton, M.D.

3

Neurology of Acquired Immune Deficiency Syndrome

Neurologic complications are estimated to occur in 30 percent of patients with acquired immune deficiency syndrome (AIDS), and in 10 percent these complications are the initial clinical problem (1, 2). Four primary disease categories are designated in AIDS by the Centers for Disease Control: *Pneumocystis carinii* pneumonia (PCP) alone, Kaposi's sarcoma (KS) alone, PCP and KS, and other opportunistic infections (3). Neurologic complications are most common in the category of other opportunistic infections. Four basic mechanisms underlie these complications: infectious, parainfectious, neoplastic, and paraneoplastic. All levels of the neuraxis can be affected; cerebral involvement is most common (4–7).

The infections or malignancies which involve the nervous system can be predicted by the cellular immune defect and are similar to those reported in immunosuppressed transplant recipients (8). B-cell malignancies, the most common neoplasms, are possibly related to Epstein-Barr virus infection (9–11). Opportunistic pathogens that may cause neurologic syndromes are listed below:

This work was partially supported by a Basic Research Grant from Columbia University.

DNA Viruses
- Herpes Group
  - Cytomegalovirus (CMV)
  - Herpes simplex virus (HSV)
  - Epstein-Barr virus (EBV)
  - Varicella-zoster virus (VZV)
- Papovavirus

Fungi
- *Filobasidiella (Cryptococcus) neoformans*
- *Aspergillus*
- *Candida albicans*

Protozoa
- *Toxoplasma gondii*

Bacteria
- *Mycobacterium avium-intracellulare* (MAI)
- *Treponema pallidum*

NEUROLOGIC ILLNESS PRESENTING AS PSYCHOPATHOLOGY

In AIDS, neurologic disease may be manifested initially by symptoms that mimic functional psychiatric syndromes. This phenomenon will be addressed briefly and illustrated by a case report before the clinical neurological complications are discussed.

Psychiatric symptoms occur most often in AIDS patients with opportunistic infections and in some patients precede other manifestations of AIDS. They may be related to systemic infection (with or without cerebral involvement), primary cerebral infection, or metabolic abnormalities. Persons who have not developed the standard criteria for a diagnosis of AIDS may complain of insomnia, anxiety, irritability, and emotional lability which interfere with work performance or personal relationships. Some describe a loss of interest in usual activities and may voluntarily withdraw from social contacts. Psychotic symptoms of paranoid delusions or severe depression may result in an evaluation by a psychiatrist or admission for psychiatric treatment. Cognitive function is normal or mildly impaired but can be difficult to assess when psychotic symptoms are present. There are no lateralizing signs on neurologic evaluation, but diffuse motor weakness or other nonfocal neurologic abnormalities may occur. The maximum interval between the onset of psychiatric symptoms and those more typical of AIDS is variable; several months are not unusual.

Psychiatric symptoms should be differentiated by the history, physical findings, and laboratory evaluation from functional psychiatric disorders and symptoms caused by brain infection.

It should be established whether the patient belongs to a group at risk for AIDS. The history should include information about sexual practices, parenteral drug use, country of origin, transfusions, and past treatment for gonorrhea, syphilis, or hepatitis. Recent or current oral candidal or genital herpes infection and unexplained constitutional, pulmonary, or gastrointestinal symptoms suggest AIDS rather than a functional disorder.

The physical examination should include a detailed neurological examination to exclude focal abnormalities that might indicate cerebral infection. The pathogens that cause cerebral infections in immunosuppressed hosts may lack features typical of encephalitis; insidious behavioral change is often the only initial symptom.

The general laboratory evaluation should include studies of metabolic parameters and the immune system as well as diagnostic studies to determine whether localized or disseminated infection or malignancy exists. Contrast-enhanced computerized tomography (CT) scan, EEG, and examination of cerebrospinal fluid (CSF) is indicated. In patients with psychiatric symptoms and a nonfocal exam, the CT scan is normal or shows cortical atrophy, the EEG is normal or shows mild to moderate nonfocal slowing; and the CSF is normal or shows a slightly elevated protein level or the presence of a few mononuclear cells.

The cause of psychiatric symptoms is uncertain but appears to be related to an associated systemic infection, most commonly due to CMV or MAI. The associated pathogen is not always readily proven at the onset of symptoms. Once documented, treatment is indicated but often ineffective. Pathologic abnormalities described in the brain are similar to those seen in viral infection and include microglial nodules, diffuse astrocytosis, and focal demyelination.

These abnormalities are sometimes insufficient to account for the clinical symptoms. In some brains, CMV inclusions or MAI are identified, but it is possible that the brain infection is a late consequence of prolonged hematogenous seeding and not the cause of the initial symptoms.

The clinical course is one of progressive physical deterioration with death usually caused by systemic infection. Mental symptoms may remain static, become exacerbated by metabolic problems, or progress to severe dementia or to a severely apathetic, negative, and withdrawn state. The latter is often erroneously thought to be dementia. Patients may remain in bed and refuse diagnostic studies, nutrition, and medical and nursing support. Careful examination is required to determine whether depression rather than dementia accounts for this behavior. The following case report illustrates a patient who presented with a syndrome that was initially thought to be psychiatric illness.

Case Report

In June 1981, a 27-year-old homosexual editor consulted a psychiatrist because he had experienced a personality change for two months. A friend of the patient reported that the patient lost his job because of hostile behavior, slovenly personal habits, and social isolation. The patient also had experienced paranoid delusions, anorexia, weight loss, and insomnia. A month earlier he had been treated for "bronchitis" and oral thrush (candidiasis), and had complained of chronic fatigue since treatment for hepatitis, gonorrhea, and syphilis two years before. The patient's psychiatric history was unremarkable; he occasionally used marijuana, intranasal cocaine, and amyl nitrite. One brother had a previous psychiatric hospitalization.

Examination revealed a thought disorder with paranoid delusions. Judgment was impaired but orientation was intact. Acute schizophrenia was diagnosed.

Two weeks later the patient was hospitalized for fever, cachexia, oral thrush, and cervical and inguinal lymphadenopathy. He remained hospitalized for six weeks, and an immune deficiency state was diagnosed. He was treated with blood transfusions, antibiotics, and antituberculous medication. There was no significant change in his behavior. Two months after discharge he spent two weeks in a psychiatric hospital for treatment of depression and recurrent oral thrush. Symptomatic improvement was brief.

Again after two months, in December 1981, the patient was hospitalized for confusion and weakness. He was alert, apathetic, paranoid, inattentive, and easily distractable. Orientation to time and place was variable. Speech was fluent and clear. He could not relate his past history, recall three objects, or perform simple calculations. Comprehension was normal for simple tasks. Naming, reading, repetition, writing, and construction were unimpaired. There was generalized muscle wasting and symmetric weakness. A mild postural tremor was present in the arms. Alternating limb movements were slow and clumsy. His gait was broad-based, unsteady, and waddling. Reflexes are symmetrically brisk with bilateral plantor flexor responses. Physical examination showed fever, cachexia, alopecia, excoriated perianal rash, oral thrush, and bilateral chorioretinitis that was worse in the left eye.

Laboratory studies showed mild anemia, leukopenia, and moderately elevated liver function tests and creatine kinase level. Transbronchial biopsy was negative for *P. carinii*. CSF examination was normal. An EEG showed generalized mild slowing, and a CT scan showed cortical atrophy.

The left eye was enucleated on January 1, 1982, because of progressive chorioretinitis with blindness; CMV necrotizing retinitis and papillitis were seen by histologic examination. Viral cultures were negative.

The patient subsequently developed fever and progressive leukopenia. Haloperidol was given for two weeks to control agitation and paranoid delusions. A single generalized seizure occurred on January 4 when his serum sodium level was 124 mEq/liter. CSF at that time showed faint oligoclonal bands. On January 5, he was alert, uncooperative, fluctuating in orientation, paranoid, and inattentive. A Parkinsonian syndrome developed that was attributed to haloperidol, which was discontinued.

Treatment with acyclovir improved the anal herpes and CMV chorioretinitis; the neurologic abnormalities seemed static. The psychotic symptoms precluded accurate assessment of memory and intellectual function, but the patient was said to converse normally with his family.

On January 31, massive gastrointestinal hemorrhage and hypoglycemia resulted in cardiac arrest. The patient died 24 hours later with refractory supraventricular tachycardia and metabolic acidosis.

Autopsy Findings. Autopsy revealed generalized atypical mycobacterial infection involving lymph nodes, spleen, liver, and testis; sepsis due to *Pseudomonas aeruginosa*; confluent necrotizing bronchopneumonia with abscess formation and associated vasculitis; focal hemorrhagic necrosis of the adrenal glands; focal chronic myocarditis; chronic erosive esophagitis and hemorrhagic gastritis; focal nephrosclerosis, bilateral; and scattered hepatocytes positive for hepatitis B surface antigen by orcein stains.

Gross examination of the patient's brain and spinal cord was normal except for slightly congested meningeal blood vessels and a small area of subarachnoid blood over the right occipital pole. Brain weight was 1260 grams. Microscopically, there were scattered microglial nodules in gray matter in the thalamus, putamen, and midbrain. In the putamen, there was a focal area of demyelination. Focally, in the tectum of the midbrain, large multinucleate cells were also found. Stains for bacteria, acid-fast bacilli, and fungi were negative. The leptomeninges of the right occipital pole contained erythrocytes without inflammatory cells consistent with agonal hemorrhage. No inclusion bodies were seen in neurons or glia. Examination of peripheral nerve and muscle by routine hematoxylin and eosin stains showed no abnormality. The right eye was not examined.

CLINICAL SYNDROMES RESULTING FROM AIDS

Infectious and Parainfectious Neurologic Complications

Meningitis. Infectious meningitis in AIDS is caused by viral, fungal, or spirochetal infection. Viral or aseptic meningitis is an

Table 1 Laboratory and Pathologic Findings in Cerebral Syndromes Caused by AIDS

Diagnosis	Cerebrospinal Fluid	Electroencephogram	Computerized Tomography	Pathology
Infectious or parainfectious				
Aseptic meningitis	↑WBC, monocytes G, normal or mild↓ ↑P, mild to moderate	NA	Normal or meningeal enhancement	NA
Cryptococcal meningitis	↑WBC, monocytes ↓G, ↑P (moderate) (all can be normal) India ink +, culture + Antigen titer +	NA	Meningeal enhancement	NA
Subacute encephalopathy	Normal findings; or ↑WBC, monocytes (rarely, PMNLs) G, normal or ↓ ↑P (usually <150)	Normal; or mild to moderate nonfocal slowing	Normal; or cortical atrophy; ventricular dilatation; white matter may appear hypodense	Microglial nodules; astrocytosis; focal white matter demyelination; associated pathogens: CMV, HSV, MAI
Toxoplasmosis	Normal findings; or ↑WBC, monocytes (usually <100) G, normal or ↓ ↑P (usually <150)	Normal; or diffuse or focal slowing	Ring-enhancing mass lesions, single or multiple (especially basal ganglia); hypodense white or gray matter lesions	Necrotic abscesses containing free trophozoites or tachyzoites in brain parenchyma, leptomeninges

Progressive multifocal leukoencephalopathy	Normal findings; or ↑P (usually <100)	Irregular moderate to severe slowing; or normal	Hypodense white matter lesions without mass effect	Multifocal demyelination with macrophage infiltration; intranuclear inclusions in oligodendroglia
Neoplastic				
Meningeal carcinomatosis	Normal findings; or ↑WBC, ↓G, ↑P cytology +	NA	Meningeal enhancement	Tumor cell infiltration in leptomeninges, basilar predominance; encasement of cranial nerve, spinal cord roots, or plexus can occur
Primary lymphoma	Normal	NA	Homogenously enhancing lesion, single (can also variably enhance or be hypodense)	Histiocytic tumor cells in brain, perivascular spaces, leptomeninges

Abbreviations: WBC = white blood cells; G = glucose; P = protein; PMNLs = polymorphonuclear leukocytes; NA = not applicable.

acute illness characterized by fever, headaches, and meningeal signs. Significant lateralizing signs and mental impairment do not occur, but cranial neuropathy may. In a series of 50 patients who had neurologic complications of AIDS, four individuals had aseptic meningitis; however, a specific viral etiology was not established (2).

Any of the herpes group of viruses may cause aseptic meningitis. A presumptive diagnosis is made by exclusion of other causes of pleocytosis in the CSF and a four-fold change in serologic titer of antibody to a specific virus. A diagnostic change in titer may not occur in immunocompromised patients. The virus is rarely recovered from CSF. No treatment is indicated since recovery is usual. Aseptic meningitis alone in a person from a risk group for AIDS should not be considered diagnostic of AIDS without confirmatory clinical or laboratory evidence.

Fungal meningitis in AIDS is usually caused by *F. neoformans* (12, 13). This organism causes a subacute or chronic meningitis and results in a depressed sensorium and cranial neuropathy more often than viral meningitis. CSF cell count and chemistries can be normal, but the diagnosis is established by demonstration of the organism in India ink smears, positive culture, and elevated antigen titer (Table 1). Treatment with amphotericin B and 5-fluorocytosine is often effective.

A history of treated syphilis is common in AIDS patients. Active meningovascular syphilis has been diagnosed in some patients on the basis of high CSF titers of reaginic and treponemal antigens; the titers normally return to normal in response to penicillin treatment. Such tests must be interpreted with caution because false-positive reaginic tests are common, the treponemal antigen tests in CSF can be unreliable, and the treponemal antibody may persist after remote infection.

Encephalitis. The clinical syndromes which accompany parenchymal cerebral infections in AIDS are distinguished by a subacute to chronic course and the frequent absence of signs suggestive of brain infection (fever, headache, and CSF pleocytosis). Insidious behavioral change is often the only initial symptom and may be mistaken for psychiatric illness. When focal signs occur, the clinical history commonly suggests neoplasm rather than infection.

Subacute Infectious or Parainfectious Encephalopathy. The most common neurologic complication in AIDS is a progressive mental change occurring in patients with opportunistic infections (2, 4). Mental signs in these patients are related to systemic infection, with or without cerebral involvement, or metabolic abnormalities. The dominant mental abnormality is either dementia with or without psychiatric features, psychiatric symptoms with or without cognitive impairment, or toxic-metabolic encephalopathy—a confusional state of inattentiveness, disorientation, and visual hallucinations.

Mental symptoms, either cognitive or psychiatric, can precede other manifestations of AIDS, or they can occur at any time during the course of the illness. Encephalopathy is more likely to occur in those with well-established disease and secondary toxic-metabolic abnormalities. Either a progressive cognitive loss or a confusional state was the most common mental change in one series (2). In some patients, however, psychiatric signs are dominant, with a clear sensorium and minimal cognitive impairment (4). Anxiety or depressive disorders are most common, but more extreme conditions such as paranoid psychosis can occur. A careful mental status examination is necessary to differentiate dementia from depression or psychosis. Generalized seizures occur in this diagnostic group but are usually related to metabolic problems.

There are no diagnostic laboratory abnormalities: CSF and CT findings are normal or nonspecific (Table 1). Multiple concurrent opportunistic infections are usually present and cause progressive physical deterioration and death. Disseminated CMV, MAI, and —in one case—HSV correlate most closely with this clinical syndrome. These pathogens can be found in postmortem brain, but abnormalities in the brain are most often nonspecific and brain infection is not documented (Table 1) (4, 7, 14–16).

There is no effective lasting treatment for disseminated CMV. Successful treatment with adenine arabinoside (ara-A) has been reported in immunocompetent patients with CMV encephalitis

(17). In the immunocompromised host, the effects of ara-A on CMV are transient. There is evidence, however, that interferons are effective in reducing both CMV-related and other herpes viral syndromes when given prophylactically in renal transplant recipients (18, 19). Treatment of MAI has been uniformly unsuccessful because of the multiple drug resistances characteristic of this organism. A new rifampicin derivative, ansamycin, is under investigational study (20).

Toxoplasmosis. *T. gondii* is a ubiquitous protozoal pathogen capable of causing either symptomatic or inapparent infection in humans that results in serologic response and latency. Favored tissue sites for latent organisms are eye, brain, or skeletal muscle. In the immunocompromised host, primary or reactivated infection often involves these target organs and may result in chorioretinitis, cerebral syndromes, or myopathy.

Cerebral toxoplasmosis is the most commonly documented focal brain infection in AIDS and is especially frequent in Haitian immigrants and parenteral drug users (2, 21). The cerebral syndromes which occur are encephalopathy without lateralizing signs, meningoencephalitis, and single or multiple mass lesions (22). The clinical course may be fulminant, with focal neurologic signs and associated headache, fever, and seizures, or insidiously progressive over weeks.

Toxoplasma chorioretinitis can occur with or without symptomatic cerebral involvement. Toxoplasma polymyositis is known to occur, but in AIDS, the relationship of this pathogen to elevation of creatine kinase levels and reported necrotizing myopathy is speculative (2, 4, 23). Viral infection and autoimmune phenomena may also cause such myopathy.

The diagnosis of toxoplasmosis is made on the basis of biopsy, serologic titers, and isolation of the organism. The diagnosis is most often established by pathologic examination of biopsy tissue. However, multiple ring-enhancing lesions on CT, which is characteristic of cerebral toxoplasmosis, and a single high titer of antibody are a reasonable basis for treatment when cerebral biopsy cannot be performed. There is less certainty about the diagnosis when a CT lesion is single. Double-dose contrast may identify other lesions when a single lesion is seen (24). A four-fold change in IgG (Sabin-Feldman) antibody titer or an elevated IgM antibody titer is required for serologic diagnosis. However, nondiagnostic IgG elevations are common in AIDS. Isolation of the organism is possible only in specialized laboratories. Treatment with pyrimethamine and sulfadiazine is usually effective.

Progressive Multifocal Leukoencephalopathy (PML). PML is a cerebral demyelinating disease caused by a papovavirus, JC virus. Demyelination is caused by the selective infection of oligodendroglial cells by this virus. Peripheral myelin is unaffected. Like *T. gondii*, JC virus is ubiquitous. By serologic studies, 70 percent of the U.S. population has evidence of prior exposure. Reactivation or primary infection occurs rarely in immunocompromised patients, including those with AIDS (2, 13, 25).

The clinical course is a subacute progressive disorder characterized by focal or multifocal neurologic signs and symptoms which localize to the cerebral hemispheres, cerebellum, or brain stem. CSF or EEG abnormalities are nonspecific; significant CSF abnormalities may indicate superinfection (Table 1). CT shows hypodense nonenhancing white matter lesions without mass effect.

The diagnosis of PML is made by brain biopsy. Antiviral therapy is usually ineffective, but remission with cytosine arabinoside has been reported (26). Because spontaneous arrest and remission can occur, the efficacy of any treatment is difficult to assess.

Other Syndromes. Candidal and bacterial brain abscesses have been reported. These organisms are usually identified in the peripheral blood or pulmonary lesions, but cerebral biopsy is required for diagnosis and appropriate treatment. VZV causes mucocutaneous lesions in AIDS and, untreated, can involve cranial nerves, arteries, brain, and spinal cord. Cerebral infarction due to VZV-related arteritis has been postulated in one patient with AIDS (2). Treatment with acyclovir arrests cutaneous zoster and lessens the risk for neurologic involvement (27). Autoimmune thrombocytopenia may be caused by CMV and may result in subarachnoid or parenchymal cerebral hemorrhage.

Retinitis in AIDS may be infectious or parainfectious (28). Ocular infection may be caused by *T. gondii*, CMV, and rarely *P. carinii*. Parainfectious retinitis is most commonly associated with systemic CMV infection and elevated levels of immune complexes in the blood. It is speculated that immune complex vasculitis is the cause.

Transverse myelopathy, Guillain-Barré syndrome, and peripheral neuropathy in AIDS are most likely related to viral infection (1, 2, 6, 7). Any of the herpesviruses can be related to these complications (29–31). Serologic titers or viral isolation are the means of establishing an etiologic diagnosis.

Neoplasms and Paraneoplastic Neurologic Complications

B-cell neoplasms are the most common malignancies that involve the nervous system in AIDS. Primary cerebral lymphoma, meningeal carcinomatosis due to systemic lymphoma, and spinal cord neoplasms are also reported (2, 11, 32). Kaposi's sarcoma is rarely metastatic to brain (33). Meningeal carcinomatosis causes cranial neuropathy, radicular pain, limb weakness, sensory loss, and areflexia. Positive CSF cytology is diagnostic but negative results may occur despite repeated examinations (2). Spinal cord neoplasms result in spinal cord signs and abnormal myelography. The diagnosis is made by surgery. Nonbacterial thrombotic endocarditis with cerebral infarction is a reported paraneoplastic complication.

LABORATORY STUDIES

Except for the characteristic T-helper lymphocyte depletion, resultant T-helper to T-suppressor cell ratio inversion and cutaneous anergy, there are no specific diagnostic laboratory findings in patients with neurologic complications. Localized or disseminated infection or malignancy is the underlying cause of neurologic syndromes. Serologic studies for hepatitis A and B antigen and antibody, *T. gondii*, and herpesviruses are indicated but may fail to confirm acute infection.

More useful for diagnosis in patients with cerebral syndromes and cranial neuropathy are contrast-enhanced CT scan, examination of CSF, and biopsy of cerebral lesions. Focal lesions on CT scan correlate with focal neurologic signs in most cases. The nature of the cerebral process may sometimes be inferred from the appearance of the CT lesion, but there is sufficient overlap to warrant biopsy when feasible (Table 1) (24, 34, 35). Biopsy is unlikely to be useful in patients with a nonfocal examination whose CT scans are normal or show cortical atrophy. CSF cell count and chemistries are nondiagnostic but smears, cultures, cytology, and cryptococcal antigen titers may establish specific diagnoses (Table 1).

Spine roentgenograms and myelography are indicated for patients with spinal cord signs. Laminectomy is required when myelography is abnormal. Surgical specimens should be cultured for bacteria, fungi, and viruses. Polyneuropathy, peripheral neuropathy, and myopathy (or elevated creatine kinase level) should be investigated by examination of CSF, electromyography and nerve conduction studies, complete metabolic screening, immune complex determinations, viral cultures, and determination of antibody titers to herpesviruses and *T. gondii*. Biopsy should be considered since the pathogenesis is obscure.

PATHOLOGY

Pathologic abnormalities in the brain may be either nonspecific or indicate a specific infection or malignancy (Table 1). Microglial nodules, astrocytosis, and focal demyelination are found in patients with subacute encephalopathy. Similar abnormalities occur in the brains of transplant recipients and are often attributed to CMV infection because CMV inclusions are occasionally found (36, 37). These changes are, however, nonspecific, and they may be caused by other pathogens or possibly be parainfectious in nature. Thus, despite the occasional finding of a major associated pathogen in the brain, such as CMV or MAI, it is uncertain whether the cerebral syndrome is always caused by infection. Because of nonspecific histopathologic changes, MAI cerebral infection may be overlooked if appropriate stains are not performed (38, 39). There is often no correlation between the severity of cerebral symptoms and the pathologic abnormalities.

Specific features of toxoplasmosis, PML, and primary or meningeal lymphoma are usually found on routine histopathology. In some cases, however, immunohistochemical studies or electron microscopy are required for the specific diagnosis.

SUMMARY

Neurologic syndromes in AIDS are related to infection or malignancy. All levels of the neuraxis can be affected, and neurologic complications may be an initial symptom of AIDS or may occur at any time during the clinical course. Aggressive evaluation, including biopsy of cerebral lesions, is needed before an appropriate treatment can be given.

References

1. Bredesen DE, Messing R: Neurological syndromes heralding the acquired immune deficiency syndrome. Ann Neurol 14:141, 1983

2. Snider WD, Simpson DM, Nielsen S, et al: Neurological complications of acquired immune deficiency syndrome: analysis of 50 patients. Ann Neurol 14:403–418, 1983

3. Centers for Disease Control: Update: acquired immune deficiency syndrome (AIDS)—United States. MMWR 32:465–467, 1983

4. Britton CB, Marquardt MD, Koppel B, et al: Neurological complications of the gay immunosuppressed syndrome: clinical and pathological features. Ann Neurol 12:80, 1982

5. Gopinatham G, Lauberstein LJ, Mondale B, et al: Central nervous system manifestations of the acquired immunodeficiency syndrome (AID) in homosexual men. Neurology (NY) 33:105, 1983

6. Herman P: Neurological complications of acquired immunologic deficiency syndrome. Neurology (NY) 33:105, 1983

7. Horowitz SL, Benson DF, Gottlieb MS, et al: Neurological complications of gay-related immunodeficiency disorder. Ann Neurol 12:80, 1982

8. Armstrong D, Wong B: Central nervous system infections in immunocompromised hosts. Ann Rev Med 33:293–308, 1982

9. Centers for Disease Control: Diffuse, undifferentiated non-Hodgkins lymphoma among homosexual males—United States. MMWR 31:277–279, 1982

10. Hochberg FH, Miller G, Schooley RT, et al: Central nervous system lymphoma related to Epstein-Barr virus. N Engl J Med 309:745–748, 1983

11. Snider WD, Simpson DM, Aronyk KE: Primary lymphoma of the nervous system associated with acquired immunodeficiency syndrome. N Engl J Med 308:45, 1983

12. Follansbee SE, Busch DF, Wofsky CB, et al: An outbreak of *Pneumocystis carinii* pneumonia in homosexual men. Ann Intern Med 96(part 1):705–713, 1982

13. Mildvan D, Mathur U, Enlow RW, et al: Opportunistic infections and immune deficiency in homosexual men. Ann Intern Med 96(part 1):700–704, 1982

14. Nielsen SL, Urmacher C, Petito CK: Encephalopathy in acquired immune deficiency syndrome (AIDS). J Neuropathol Exp Neurol 42:326, 1983

15. Sohn CC, Schroff RW, Kliewer KE, et al: Disseminated *Mycobacterium avium-intracellulare* infection in homosexual men with

acquired cell-mediated immunodeficiency: a histologic and immunologic study of two cases. Am J Clin Pathol 79:247–252, 1983

16. Zakowski P, Fligiel S, Berlin OGW, et al: Disseminated *Mycobacterium avium-intracellulare* infection in homosexual men dying of acquired immunodeficiency. JAMA 248:2980–2982, 1982

17. Phillips CA, Fanning WL, Gump DW, et al: Cytomegalovirus encephalitis in immunologically normal adults: successful treatment with vidarabine. JAMA 238:2299–2300, 1977

18. Cheeseman SH, Rubin RH, Stewart JA, et al: Controlled clinical trial of prophylactic human leukocyte interferon in renal transplantation: effects on cytomegalovirus and herpes simplex virus infections. N Engl J Med 300: 1345–1349, 1979

19. Hirsch MS, Schooley RT, Cosimi B, et al: Effects of interferon-alpha on cytomegalovirus reactivation syndromes in renal-transplant recipients. N Engl J Med 308:1489–1493, 1983

20. FDA Bulletin 12:22, 1982

21. Hauser WE, Luft BJ, Conley FK, et al: Central nervous system toxoplasmosis in homosexual and heterosexual adults. N Engl J Med 307:498–499, 1982

22. Townsend JJ, Wolinsky TS, Baringer TR, et al: Acquired toxoplasmosis. Arch Neurol 32:335–343, 1975

23. Rowland LP, Greer M: Toxoplasmic polymyositis. Neurology 11:367–370, 1961

24. Post MJD, Chan JC, Hemsley GT, et al: Toxoplasma encephalitis in Haitian adults with acquired immunodeficiency syndrome: a clinical pathologic CT correlation. American Journal of Roentgenology 140:861–868, 1983

25. Miller JR, Barrett RE, Britton CB, et al: Progressive multifocal leukoencephalopathy in a male homosexual with T-cell immune deficiency. N Engl J Med 307:1436–1438, 1982

26. Marriott PJ, O'Brien MD, Mackenzie CK, et al: Progressive multifocal leukoencephalopathy: remission with cytarabine. J Neurol Neurosurg Psychiatry 38:205–209, 1975

27. Balfour AH, Bean B, Laskin O, et al: Acyclovir halts progression of herpes zoster in immunocompromised patients. N Engl J Med 308:1448–1453, 1983

28. Holland GN, Gottlieb MS, Yec RD, et al: Ocular disorders associated with a new severe acquired immunodeficiency syndrome. Am J Ophthalmol 93:393–402, 1982

29. Hogan EL, Krigman MR: Herpes zoster myelitis. Arch Neurol 29:309–313, 1973

30. Klastersky J, Cappel R, Snoeck JM, et al: Ascending myelitis in association with herpes-simplex virus. N Engl J Med 287:182–184, 1972

31. Kleemola E, Wechman N, Haltia K, et al: The Guillain-Barré syndrome associated with acquired cytomegalovirus infection. Acta Med Scand 181:603–607, 1967

32. Pitchenik AE, Fischl MA, Walls KW: Evaluation of cerebral-mass lesions in acquired immunodeficiency syndrome. N Engl J Med 308:1099, 1983

33. Hymes KB, Greene JB, Marcus A, et al: Kaposi's sarcoma in homosexual men—a report of eight cases. Lancet 2:598–600, 1981

34. Enzmann DR, Brant-Zawadski M, Britt RH: CT of the central nervous system infections in immunocompromised patients. American Journal of Roentgenology 135:263–267, 1980

35. Tadmor R, Davis KA, Robinson GH, et al: CT in primary malignant lymphoma of the brain (reticulum cell). J Comput Assist Tomogr 2:135–140, 1978

36. Dorfman LJ: Cytomegalovirus encephalopathy in adults. Neurology (Minneapolis) 23:136–144, 1973

37. Schneck SA: Neuropathological features of human organ transplantation, I: probable cytomegalovirus infection. J Neuropathol Exp Neurol 24:415–429, 1965

38. Cohen RJ, Samosznk MK, Busch D, et al: Occult infections with *Mycobacterium intracellulare* in bone marrow specimens from patients with AIDS. N Engl J Med 308:1475, 1983

39. Greene JE, Sidhu GS, Lewis S, et al: *Mycobacterium avium-intracellulare*: a cause of life-threatening infection in homosexuals and drug abusers. Ann Intern Med 97:539–546, 1982

PSYCHIATRIC TREATMENT

This section presents the findings of four individuals who have had extensive experience in psychiatric assistance to persons affected by AIDS: patients, their friends and loved ones, and their families. Each paper has a different focus. Dr. Forstein begins with a presentation of a conceptual framework that is helpful in approaching persons who do not have the disease but are excessively anxious about it. Dr. Dilley outlines the issues and techniques helpful with diagnosed AIDS patients. Dr. Barbuto discusses the treatment of psychiatric complications in patients with advanced disease, and Dr. Nichols presents an overview of the role of two special types of group therapy. Readers are again reminded that neurological complications in persons with AIDS may present as functional psychiatric illness. There is also the possibility that patients with advanced AIDS, who frequently receive numerous experimental drugs, may develop side effects that resemble a depressive or psychotic disorder.

There is admittedly some redundancy here and in the next section. Lillian Hellman has brought to our attention the value of pentimento, and the overlapping in this monograph offers us an opportunity to view the various shades with which each author chooses to color his or her picture of AIDS. This seems to be the best representation of the state of the art; the complex portrait of AIDS is just now beginning to emerge.

There is advice and guidance here for mental health professionals who are called upon to counsel persons who have or who are concerned about AIDS. There are also many areas where there are still more questions than answers. Imaginative and innovative solutions to clinical problems are also presented for which both psychiatry and the involved community groups deserve credit. The ultimate responsibility of psychiatrists treating AIDS patients is to ensure that they receive dignified and sympathetic treatment and that their reasonable wishes are respected, even if, at times, these desires conflict with the "wisest" medical course.

4

AIDS Anxiety in the "Worried Well"

Marshall Forstein, M.D.

AIDS Anxiety in the "Worried Well"

The psychological syndromes associated with the acquired immune deficiency syndrome (AIDS) are multifaceted and complex. Persons with AIDS are prone to develop a variety of psychiatric conditions, organic and psychogenic, which may vary as the illness relentlessly continues: these are described elsewhere. In addition, there are clinical syndromes recognizable in persons who have been called the "worried well" (those who do not have AIDS) and the "walking wounded" (those who may have an early form of the syndrome but do not meet present diagnostic criteria).

AIDS anxiety, Kaposi's neurosis, and AIDS phobia are terms that have been used in the lay press to describe the psychological impact of AIDS. This chapter will attempt to provide a conceptual framework for evaluating and treating people who suffer psychologically from the existence and potential threat of that catastrophic illness.

In so doing, it is imperative to distinguish, both theoretically and clinically, between anxiety and fear. In this regard, Campbell's *Psychiatric Dictionary* (1) is helpful. It states, "Fear is a reaction to a real or threatened danger, while anxiety is more typically a reaction to an unreal or imagined danger." Campbell also points out that fear lacks two characteristics of anxiety: "an apprehensive self-absorption which interferes with an effective and advantageous solution of reality problems," and "an irresolvable doubt concerning the nature, . . . the actual appearance, . . . and the best objective means of reducing or removing the evil. . . ." Campbell also reminds us that, in addition to the psychological effects, anxiety has "a somatic, psychological side (disturbed breathing, increased heart activity, vasomotor changes, and musculoskeletal disturbances such as trembling or paralysis, increased sweating, etc.)."

In considering whether there is a real danger (AIDS fear) or an unreal, imagined threat (AIDS anxiety), two questions are crucial: Is the perception of danger the same, or similar to, that of more informed and objective observers? Is the response reasonable, psychologically and behaviorally, given the available data?

Clinically, the people on whom AIDS impacts psychologically can be separated into five categories: 1) persons with nonspecific symptomatology; 2) persons with an intimate exposure to someone with AIDS; 3) persons with no known intimate exposure to someone with AIDS, but who are at some risk because of past or present sexual activity or intravenous drug use; 4) persons in the process of "coming out"; and 5) persons not at risk who incorporate anxiety about AIDS into a preexisting psychiatric disorder. It should be noted that persons concerned about AIDS may fall into more than one of the above categories.

PERSONS WITH NONSPECIFIC SYMPTOMATOLOGY

Included here are those persons who have clinical signs and symptoms of what has been called by various names, including "the diffuse lymphadenopathy syndrome," "pre-AIDS," "lesser AIDS," and the "AIDS-related complex" (ARC). The spectrum of these conditions ranges from mild symptomatology to debilitating illnesses that do not meet the CDC case definition for AIDS. The recent isolation and characterization of HTLV III virus (human T cell lymphotrophic virus, type III) supports the likelihood that AIDS and at least some cases of ARC are caused by this virus, with unknown factors determining the clinical picture. It is impossible, as of now, to predict which persons with ARC will develop AIDS. Although the discovery of HTLV III instills hope for the eventual development of a vaccine and a cure for the immunological defect, the role of this virus in AIDS is as yet so poorly understood that it adds to confusion about the syndrome. In some cases the questions raised by the announced isolation of HTLV III have produced distress in persons with AIDS or ARC. The virus may have been discovered too late to benefit those now suffering with AIDS. Testing for the virus or antibodies to it may actually increase the individual's anxiety and real fear of AIDS.

Persons with nonspecific symptomatology are difficult to treat because the symptoms are constant reminders to them that they are at risk and that some may even have an early form of the illness. Many of these persons utilize health services continuously in their ongoing need to check their health. It is often difficult to differentiate between real symptoms and the hypochondriacal aspects of their reactions. At this time, testing for HTLV III and its antibodies remains a research tool. Demands by anxious patients for services that are not yet available is likely to increase stress in health care providers who already feel limited in their capacity to intervene therapeutically.

Such patients may be helped to manage anxiety through group or individual psychotherapy, and the relationship with their primary physician is of major importance. They need a reassuring, calm, and stabilizing posture from their health care providers, both medical and psychologic. Above all, the person's fear of abandonment must be turned aside through a realistic discussion of the limitations of the therapy. Some patients will visit physicians every day, often with the same question as the day before; the emotional shock of AIDS can distort communication drastically. Patients can overwhelm physicians who do not utilize community services to augment their care.

In addition, doctors should take a thorough sexual history with a detailed review of sexual practices and experience. A thorough history of drug use should also be obtained. Only by so doing can reasonable assessments of risk be made and appropriate recommendations be given. Physicians must be able to put aside any personal feelings they may have about the sexual or drug-related behavior of patients; any negative bias on the part of the therapist will be picked up by patients and will add to their distress. There is need for sophistication as well as practicality. For example, asking patients to give up sex entirely is a useless and futile prospect. Some patients do choose this option, but usually temporarily. A mutual and frank exploration of sexual practices oriented specifically to the likelihood of transmitting pathogens is more helpful. Such a discussion will often allow the patient to trade off one practice for another that is less dangerous, one with the attendant perception of compromise. Sometimes the cessation of previously enjoyed pleasures will be accompanied by mourning and will be regarded as a self-imposed loss until such time when AIDS is no longer a threat to life.

Close liaison should be maintained between the providers of medical and psychiatric care. Persons with excessive anxiety may require encouragement by therapists to see their primary physicians about physical problems. Psychiatrists can assist the medical team by coordinating anxiety-reducing modalities, suggesting pharmacologic intervention, and assessing the need for ongoing therapy. Psychiatric consultation is indicated for those individuals who show either excessive or inappropriately diminished concern about AIDS. Internists should report any change in AIDS patients' physical condition to psychotherapists.

The presence of physiological signs sometimes creates such anxiety that pharmacological intervention with antianxiety agents is essential. Without medication patients may experience an acute regression to a helpless state which may include suicidal ideation. There is beginning to be evidence that a decrease in exposure to transmissible pathogens, through changes in sexual behavior or the use of drugs, may prevent the inexorable progression to full-blown AIDS. Therefore, supportive therapy for such persons should emphasize the types of changes that will reduce the real risks to the individual's health. A reduction in anxiety should also ensue.

PERSONS WITH AN INTIMATE EXPOSURE TO SOMEONE WITH AIDS

The first and second categories of potential patients are qualitatively different from the others in that there is a real likelihood that persons in these categories may have come in contact with the cause of AIDS. Some of these people may become hysterical and panicky, or even delusional in believing they have the disease. Those with extended contact who have not developed symptoms may develop a sense of being immune to AIDS, and may act with one of several postures. Some proceed to live as before. Others, concerned that they might harbor the putative AIDS agent, restrict their intimate contacts out of a sense of moral responsibility. Still others develop a survivor's guilt and may become more active sexually or become depressed and guilt-ridden.

To determine whether an exposed individual's response is appropriate, several questions may be asked. Has there been a single contact, or has the exposure been multiple or repeated? Has the person had physiological signs or symptoms which might account, at least in part, for his fear? What underlying emotional supports are available to him? Can the person deal with the inevitable anger towards the person who exposed him to AIDS? This is particularly problematic if the person is dying. Is that person someone he loves or a casual sex partner?

To the extent that persons feel safe, or feel infected and tentative about life, they will exhibit various patterns of social interaction. Some gay men, for example, integrate the crisis into their lives and participate in individual or community efforts to control the epidemic. For others it is a time of social withdrawal and negative self-identification, rejecting the homosexual community which has been blamed for the illness. Drug addicts and Haitians often do not have this choice; addicts have no organized response to AIDS, whereas Haitians may find themselves rejected by their own established community.

PERSONS WITHOUT A KNOWN EXPOSURE TO SOMEONE WITH AIDS

The third category involves persons who are at risk for AIDS because of past or present sexual activity or intravenous drug use. However, the degree of risk cannot be determined for any individual and this adds to the anxiety. Clinically, members of this group often exhibit denial, which serves to bind the anxiety. A few individuals increase risk-taking behavior, becoming more active sexually or using drugs more frequently. Others, especially those with internalized homophobia and ambivalent object relations, may present a picture of guilt with self-hate and self-recriminations. Although powerful, denial is a primitive defense that often breaks down dramatically when AIDS is diagnosed in a friend or acquaintance.

In addition, then, to the acknowledgment of real fear, some individuals develop an anxiety state characterized by the sense of powerlessness over what is seen as the inevitable destruction of the self. The physiological components of the anxiety, such as somatic pain and hyperarousal of the autonomic nervous system, serve to reinforce the patients' irresolvable doubts. All this combines to undermine the patient's ability to cope with his situation.

Again, now that the putative etiologic agent, HTLV III, has been identified and the capacity to test for the presence of that virus and antibodies to it has been developed, more questions without answers have been raised. Persons concerned about AIDS must continue to live with ambiguity and uncertainty until such time when the testing for HTLV III is standardized and readily available. Not until then will clinicians be able to determine whether an individual has been exposed to the putative agent or, more importantly, whether the individual is vulnerable to or is harboring the virus. Therefore the treatment of someone with appropriate fear and concomitant anxiety is based on helping him to maximize control over his own life, making reasonable and appropriate behavioral changes to reduce the perceived risk. For those with panic disorder or somatic symptoms of anxiety, appropriate pharmacologic intervention may help to dispel the feeling of being sick. This may allow persons to assess their situation more realistically and to mobilize or learn appropriate coping strategies.

Cognitive therapy is also effective. It can teach people to recognize the difference between fear and anxiety and help them to judge the degree of risk involved in specific sexual behaviors. The possibility that one has been exposed already cannot be dismissed for most persons; however, individuals can learn to focus on managing their present lives rather than being obsessed about the irrevocable past. This shift makes them feel that they are more in control of their destiny, increases their self-esteem, and promotes a healthier attitude about sexuality. Personality strengths and coping capacities, of course, will affect the ability to concentrate on the present rather than the past. Some patients will revert to religious tenets of their childhood with the judgment that AIDS is just retribution for their homosexual acts. Others, with less ego organization, may be overwhelmed by anxiety and, as in the first category, may become frankly hysterical or paranoid regarding the illness.

The capacity to bind anxiety and negotiate one's daily life amidst existing real dangers will fluctuate depending on existing supports and psychological concerns. The majority of gay men have responded appropriately to the fear of AIDS by creating new attitudes and experiences of social interaction among themselves. Intimacy is no longer seen as being primarily sexual. Many men, in fact, incorporate the realistic fear of AIDS into their social and intimate lives, and use it to motivate them to achieve more lasting needs and satisfactions than sexual arousal. On the other hand, as in other groups, some gay men have difficulty with nonsexual intimacy by virtue of their personality organization and the level of their object relations maturity. They find that sexual activity, which previously served to bind anxiety, is now in itself anxiety producing. Psychological issues for this group are more complex than the assessment of sexual risk. Group therapy for compulsive sexuality can promote an understanding of the sexual behavior while addressing the fears of intimacy, but some individuals are unable to commit themselves to such therapy because they fear the group process more than AIDS itself. Clearly, the anxiety over AIDS can often be simply a focal point for more deeply rooted anxieties concerning intimacy, sexuality, and the capacity to see oneself as being in control of one's life.

PERSONS IN THE PROCESS OF "COMING OUT"

AIDS has psychological effects upon persons who are "coming out" (the process of discovering, accepting, and integrating one's own homosexuality). Traditionally, sexual activity reinforces self-identification at this time, but with AIDS the fear of sex may distort or abort the process. While some gay men come out with relatively few sexual relationships before coupling, others experience more sexual activity than may now be deemed safe for health reasons. At present, because of the influence of AIDS, people just coming out should benefit from information regarding safe sex, allowing them to develop positive attitudes toward it. They also need assistance in learning of nonsexual ways to form a gay identity. How many homosexually oriented men have chosen not to come out because of AIDS is unknown, but working with gay men who began the process and were put off by the AIDS crisis suggests that it is a clinically significant issue. Since gay liberation, coming out had been facilitated by the presence of positive role models and a less hostile environment, but AIDS has again complicated the process with its negative message about sexual exploration.

PERSONS WITH A PREEXISTING PSYCHIATRIC DISORDER

The fourth category is composed of persons in whom preexisting pyschiatric conditions become infused with concern about AIDS. Whether or not they are homosexual, persons with various mental disorders may present with anxiety over AIDS as a manifest symptom. Those with an acute or chronic psychosis may develop paranoid delusions about sexual activity, sharing foodstuffs, or cohabitating. Aiding these people to understand what their past risks have been and what kinds of behavior they may safely engage in may help, but since their anxiety is caused primarily by the underlying illness, treatment must focus on it.

In people vulnerable to affective disorders, AIDS may precipitate a major depression or exacerbate the tendency toward isolation and social withdrawal. There have been cases of panic disorders being brought on by AIDS. Persons with major sexual dysfunctions may use AIDS to avoid addressing underlying concerns about intimacy and sexuality. People prone to alcohol or substance abuse may use the AIDS crisis to rationalize and support their abusive behavior. Treating the major psychopathology is essential before the AIDS anxiety can be addressed in a therapeutic manner. Unless such patients can achieve abstinence, however, treatment is likely to be unsuccessful. Temporary pharmacological intervention or hospitalization may be helpful.

Various personality disorders can present with AIDS anxiety as a prominent symptom also. People with an hysterical personality organization have been observed to use AIDS as a diversion from coping with their underlying conflicts. Persons with schizoid disorders may use the AIDS anxiety to justify withdrawal and isolation. Those with passive-dependent personalities may continue in destructive relationships, telling themselves that they fear being alone and at risk for AIDS. Those with obsessive-compulsive personalities may incorporate the concern about AIDS in a variety of ways, including obsessions about health and sexual behavior and compulsive hand-washing.

In addition, persons who have exhibited phobic responses to stress in the past may react to AIDS by becoming phobic about sex, cleanliness, and contact with people in general. Treatment of this phobia may be difficult because, again, it is always possible that the person may be, or may have been, exposed to the causative agent. Desensitization techniques are of limited value because the increase in the number and visibility of cases can counteract its effect. The use of monoamine oxidase inhibitors and benzodiazepines has been of some help.

SOCIETAL REACTIONS

It is important that mental health professionals understand the pattern of reaction to AIDS to assist individuals and communities to adjust to it in an appropriate and constructive manner. When AIDS first appears in a community, people are interested primarily in increasing their own safety. This can result in responsible changes in personal and community behavior or the irresponsible and ineffective blaming of gays and addicts for the disease, with attendant calls for quarantine and other measures that abridge their civil rights. Psychiatrists must address the prejudicial aspects of such a community reaction which, if not aborted, will increase the sense of panic and waste valuable energy needed to meet the threat. With time, most people continue to respond to AIDS in a reasonable and responsible, if less intensive, way, but there seems to be an emerging pattern that those who initially are the most hysterical are later unable to maintain an appropriate level of concern about its real dangers. Therefore, it is even more essential that psychiatrists attempt to ameliorate the initial panic when AIDS is found in an individual or community.

On a larger scale, societal response patterns indicate that the initial high level of anxiety that AIDS provokes cannot be maintained and is superseded by a relative loss of interest in the disease and even complacency toward it. Intense anxiety expends a great amount of energy, and individuals are soon exhausted by it. It is replaced, for most people, by a combination of partial acceptance and partial denial that allows for more flexibility in coping with the crisis. At this point, too much denial can lead to an irresponsible and dangerous return to pre-AIDS behavior.

SUMMARY

It is imperative, therefore, that a thorough assessment be made of anyone who presents himself for treatment because of anxiety about AIDS. It is important to uncover any preexisting psychiatric disorder and to address it vigorously in the overall treatment plan. Individual or group psychotherapy may alleviate anxiety by assisting patients to respond to AIDS in a reasonable manner, to institute more appropriate coping devices, and to change their behavior in ways that reduce their risk of contracting it. Therapists need to appreciate how different sexual identities and personality organizations may affect the individual's reaction to AIDS. Persons who have fixed delusions that they have been infected and are waiting for the disease to manifest itself are difficult to work with, as are those with so much internalized self-loathing that AIDS becomes a natural component of their negative self-image.

The general goals of treatment are to help people to recognize the control they can exercise over their lives, to let go of their feelings about the past, and to deal with their anxiety, anger, and sense of loss from this threat to their well being.

Persons in all the risk groups for AIDS (gays, addicts, Haitians, and hemophiliacs) encounter problems in their relationship with health care providers. Psychiatrists should understand that feelings of being helpless, alienated, and unempowered to make changes in their lives may have to be dealt with before therapy can be successful. Psychiatrists who retain even subtle biases toward gays, blacks, or addicts are apt to harm persons with AIDS anxiety by reinforcing negative self-concepts. In dealing with AIDS anxiety the therapist will address the person's basic concept of self-worth, his sense of power and control over his life, and his feelings about whether it is OK to be who he is and whether people like him are allowed to be powerful in our society. AIDS anxiety will diminish as an individual is able to construct a strong, positive, and realistic sense of self. AIDS will continue to elicit fear in persons at risk until it is understood, preventable, and treatable. However, with proper therapy and with a reasonable societal response, it should not cause disabling anxiety.

Reference

1. Campbell RJ: Psychiatric Dictionary, 5th ed. New York, Oxford University Press, 1981

5

Treatment Interventions and Approaches to Care of Patients with Acquired Immune Deficiency Syndrome

James W. Dilley, M.D.

5

Treatment Interventions and Approaches to Care of Patients with Acquired Immune Deficiency Syndrome

The profound medical morbidity and mortality of the acquired immune deficiency syndrome (AIDS) is by now well known. Concurrent with the physical sequelae of the syndrome is the psychological morbidity experienced both by persons with AIDS as well as those who feel themselves to be at risk of contracting the illness. This is especially true for members of the risk groups, and the mental health practitioner may be asked to intervene with those who are at risk as well as those who are already ill. Thus, there are at least three broad groups of individuals who may request services from a mental health practitioner: 1) the "worried well"—sexually active gay men who are frightened by the possibility of contracting the illness; 2) persons with AIDS-related complex—individuals who do not have a diagnosis of AIDS but have one or more nonspecific symptoms, such as lymphadenopathy, unexplained fevers, or weight loss (thought to number three to five thousand persons in San Francisco alone [1]); and 3) persons with AIDS—those with lesions of Kaposi's sarcoma or one or more of the opportunistic infections characteristic of the syndrome.

It is easy to see how individuals in each of these groups might request psychological services. However, the content of these services should differ according to an individual's needs and to those of the group to which he belongs. It is also likely that discrete subpopulations exist within the larger groups and that each may have differing needs. Consequently, different treatment approaches are appropriate.

I would like to turn to a consideration of subgroups noted among persons with AIDS and briefly explore some of the physical and psychosocial stressors these patients encounter. Later, I will explore possible treatment strategies in working with patients from the different subgroups. More extensive discussion of treatment strategies for the worried well and those with AIDS-related complexes is included in other chapters in this monograph.

To appreciate different subpopulations of AIDS patients from a psychological point of view, it is important to have an understanding of the common medical course of the illness. Though exceptions may exist, the most common course is the intermittent development of illnesses that are not usually seen among the general public. Sometimes these intermittent illnesses can be treated, leaving the patient with the underlying immune deficiency but alleviating the current illness. Subsequently, the patient may show no observable signs of illness other than easy fatigability. Sometimes the intercurrent illness can only be treated symptomatically. For example, an AIDS patient who has diarrhea because of a *Cryptosporidium* infection may be given Lomotil (diphenoxylate hydrochloride with atrophine sulfate) to improve the diarrhea, but no treatment exists for the eradication of the cryptosporidia. Thus, the patient must learn to cope with the diarrhea. For others—for example, those with Kaposi's sarcoma—who elect to be treated with interferon, there is the ongoing physical trauma of treatment. Some patients respond well, but they must learn to live with and accept the side effects of treatment—high fevers and malaise. The treatments are given frequently, three times or more per week, leading one patient to state that he was "surviving . . . for what? To stay at home feeling sick and lying on the couch all day?" Finally, as a consequence of repeated infections or the spread of Kaposi's sarcoma, the patient may weaken and die.

In addition to an appreciation for the medical complications of

AIDS, a word should be said about the social factors that make coping with the syndrome particularly difficult. From early epidemiologic reports, homosexual men with AIDS were seen as having had numerous sexual contacts, of having lived "in the fast lane" with frequent use of drug and alcohol, or of being intravenous drug users. This stereotype allows others to make assumptions about an individual's lifestyle, and thus a gay man with a diagnosis of AIDS must deal with others' reactions to the stereotype as well as to the fact of his being ill. Consequently, the reactions of friends, family members, or professionals are sometimes problematic. For some patients the diagnosis of AIDS has resulted in having to reveal their homosexuality to their families for the first time, while in others earlier conflicts over their lifestyle have been rekindled. This sense of stigma which many of the patients report also enhances the feeling for some that their sexual orientation is to blame for their illness. Self-esteem is then further compromised at a time when the patient is already struggling with the diagnosis of a life-threatening illness.

Finally, the uncertainty that surrounds all aspects of the illness, the social isolation that many patients have experienced, and the tendency of some patients to experience the illness as retribution for past behavior contributes to their difficulty in coping (2).

TREATMENT APPROACHES

I have described some of the physical and psychosocial consequences of AIDS because of the link between these factors and the psychological needs of these patients. In addition to the usual factors such as personality style, history, and the degree of social supports available to the patient, treatment approaches must also consider the medical status of the patient. Different issues will be highlighted at different points along the continuum of the illness and, consequently, different treatment approaches will need to be emphasized. With consideration of these factors, I would now like to focus on possible treatment approaches in working with diagnosed AIDS patients.

There are three general levels of care required by persons with

AIDS who are referred for psychiatric consultation. The first level of intervention is for those having few psychiatric symptoms prior to the diagnosis of AIDS who ask to talk to someone. Sometimes these persons will be referred by the primary physician because of a concern that the patient's reaction to the diagnosis is inappropriate: either the patient appears affectively overwhelmed or almost nonchalant. Such patients are best characterized as exhibiting a stress response syndrome. Once this is understood, the consultant can begin working with the patient while educating the primary physician about the nature of this reaction.

The types and patterns of psychological response to an acutely stressful event, such as the diagnosis of AIDS, have been summarized by Horowitz (3). When confronted with a traumatic event, an individual usually responds with an affective outcry, affective numbing, or unbidden thoughts or images spawned by the event that keep him in a continual state of anxiety. Many AIDS patients report intrusive thoughts of suffering and death. Commonly, patients will vascillate among these states. It is important for the consultant to keep in mind that these initial reactions probably serve an adaptive function in helping the individual fend off too-painful affects, while moving toward cognitive and affective integration of the event. This process has been termed affective completion by Lindemann (4).

As these stages likely represent adaptive defenses, it is important that the consultant not approach the individual with a bias toward affective discharge and away from cognitive denial. It may take several meetings for the patient to gradually achieve affective integration without being overwhelmed, and this process should be supported by the consultant. At times antianxiety and antidepressant medications are important; the reader is referred to a review of the considerations in the diagnosis of depression in the medically ill (5).

Once affective integration of the diagnosis occurs, at least partial control of the acute anxiety and dysphoria is achieved. The patient's focus now turns to other issues. The need for education about the illness and the possible reactions he may encounter from others; how and what to tell family members, friends, and employers; the need for ongoing emotional support; and financial planning are all at the forefront. Assertiveness training may be helpful in providing the patient with skills to secure help and support from others. Decisions regarding the use of free time and staving off boredom are issues for many as they are either unable or not allowed to continue working. Concerns regarding infectious contamination of others, both in living arrangements and in terms of possibly continued sexual activity, are common and need to be addressed. A frank discussion about alternative approaches to sexuality that do not involve the exchange of body fluids, such as mutual masturbation, the use of condoms, or the use of erotica, is helpful. Feelings of guilt on the part of the patient and the desire to blame himself for the illness need to be addressed and explored. Connections between sexual orientation and the illness should be actively challenged by pointing out the existence of the disease in other groups and discussing the difference between association and causation.

Support of psychological defenses such as altruism and denial is also useful during this early period. Encouraging the patient to become involved in altruistic activities is helpful, as this involvement enhances self-esteem and provides a meaningful outlet for the patient's remaining energies. Self-help groups, political action groups, and involvement in research projects are examples of altruistic activities.

In self-help groups, the patient not only derives support from the group but is also given the opportunity to be of help to others. This fosters an improved sense of self-esteem as well as confronting the patient's view of himself as helpless. The group also serves to reduce social isolation, and the consultant can encourage socialization and interaction among the members outside of the group.

Other patients prefer to become involved in or form political action groups. These groups work to educate the public about AIDS and the needs of AIDS patients. In major cities these groups have been successful in working with the public health system to design and implement services for AIDS patients. They have also held several successful fund raisers, with the money raised at these functions going to support programs for patients with AIDS.

Finally, many patients derive satisfaction from participating in research projects. An attitude frequently expressed is that by participating in research, new information may be discovered and "maybe some good can come from my being sick."

Supporting "denial" may also be adaptive. Earlier writers have found that patients facing terminal illness who are successful "deniers" not only lower their anxiety and raise their hopes, but also survive significantly longer (6–8). A successful "denier" may also be thought of as one who "accepts" his illness. The consultant, while acknowledging the seriousness of the illness, can facilitate this process by communicating his belief that the patient can recuperate to a level of functioning that will allow him to continue being productive. Emphatically pointing out others who have continued to engage in meaningful activity is often helpful, giving the patient hope and countering the idea that with the diagnosis of AIDS the patient's life is over. Also, if permission can be obtained from both parties, arranging a meeting between those who are successfully managing their illness with those who are newly diagnosed can be extremely helpful. Thus, individuals who acknowledge their disease, comply with medical treatment, and are able to accommodate to their illness while maintaining an active life seem to cope most effectively.

Other important treatment strategies for this group include relaxation training, hypnosis, and visualization. Visualization is a process of guided imagery in which the patient learns to see himself as healthy and disease free. The involvement of other patients with AIDS and/or gay community groups is especially helpful in maintaining the patient's self-esteem and reducing his sense of isolation.

For patients at a midstage in the disease process—for example, those hospitalized with a second bout of *Pneumocystis carinii* pneumonia or another AIDS-related infection—the focus of treatment often begins to change. Loss of hope and emotional exhaustion are often encountered. The ability of the patient to continue denying his illness is lessened, and frequently he begins to engage in more detailed grief work. The consultant encourages ventilation of feeling as the patient anticipates and mourns the multiple losses of important people and objects.

Frequently the patient begins a life review, at times focusing on a particular problematic relationship or experience. Sometimes he seeks encouragement to deal with a particularly troublesome issue in his life as he begins to think more specifically about dying. He may want to discuss issues related to the extent of treatment: what his wishes are regarding intubation, resuscitation, etc. He may need or want to write a will as well as consider appointing someone with power of attorney should he become unable to make decisions for himself. He may want to begin discussing plans for a funeral or memorial service. The consultant encourages and supports this process, taking cues from the patient and communicating to him that these are not frightful or morbid topics and that it is useful to explore them. He also provides support to family members or friends when appropriate.

The final group of AIDS patients the psychiatric consultant may be asked to see are those admitted for terminal care. In these cases, treatment is supportive and often involves working with family and friends as well as with the patient. Treatment consists largely of reassuring the patient that he will not be abandoned, and that he will be given adequate pain medication. The use of antidepressants as an adjunct to pain management is sometimes indicated. Often the patient will begin to withdraw emotional investment in others as he begins to turn away from the living and focus more on himself and his approaching death. Understanding this as a common development and communicating this to family and friends can often be very comforting to them. Furthermore, the patient is often relieved by the opportunity to discuss his fears and concerns about dying with the consultant. He is encouraged to take care of any business he feels is left to finish, is supported in his decisions regarding treatment, and ultimately may be given permission to let go of life with the understanding that the consultant will do all he can to see that the patient's wishes are followed after his death.

DISCUSSION

AIDS is a syndrome with profound medical and psychosocial consequences. When a person with AIDS has either been referred for or has requested psychiatric intervention, the consultant should bear in mind the relationship between the patient's presenting complaints and his medical status. The consultant should also be aware that in a series of psychiatric consultations with AIDS patients, the management of mood disorders and dementia are the most frequent reasons for consultation (9). For those patients with a major psychiatric diagnosis, such as major depression or dementia, standard psychiatric interventions are appropriate. Medications will play an important role, and psychotherapy will be essential for the depressed group. For those without a primary diagnosis, a consideration of the patient's medical status will be helpful. Viewing the illness as a continuum, with certain common experiences and challenges to be mastered, has proved useful in planning a treatment strategy and may involve one or more of the approaches mentioned above.

References

1. AIDS Activity Office: AIDS Mental Health Proposal. Unpublished. San Francisco, San Francisco Department of Health, 1983

2. Dilley JW, Ochitill H, Perl M, et al: Psychiatric consultation with AIDS patients. Manuscript submitted for publication

3. Horowitz MJ: Stress Response Syndromes. New York, Jason Aronson, 1976

4. Lindemann E: Symptomatology and management of acute grief. Am J Psychiatry 101:141–149, 1944

5. Cavanaugh S, Clark D, Gibbons R: Diagnosing depression in the hospitalized medically ill. Psychosomatics 24:809–815, 1983

6. Hackett TP, Weisman AD: Denial as a social factor in patients with heart disease and cancer. Ann NY Acad Sci 164:802–817, 1969

7. Hackett TP, Cassem NH: Psychological reactions to life-threatening illness, in Psychological Aspects of Stress. Edited by Abram H. Springfield, Ill, Charles C Thomas, 1970

8. Weisman AD, Hackett TP: Denial as a social act, in Creativity, Reminiscing and Dying. Edited by Leven S, Kahana R. New York, International Universities Press, 1966

9. Dilley JW, Ochitill H, Perl M, et al: Psychiatric consultations with AIDS patients. Manuscript submitted for publication

6

Psychiatric Care of Seriously Ill Patients with Acquired Immune Deficiency Syndrome

Joseph Barbuto, M.D.

6

Psychiatric Care of Seriously Ill Patients with Acquired Immune Deficiency Syndrome

In a group of young men with acquired immune deficiency syndrome (AIDS), primarily Kaposi's sarcoma (KS), seen by the Psychiatry Service of the Memorial Sloan Kettering Medical Center, certain psychological and social issues have emerged. First of all, the patient population is mature, socially aware, and highly intelligent. More than any other population of cancer patients, this one suffers a dramatic change in self-esteem, daily habits, and general lifestyle in response to the illness. They suffer from feelings of isolation, a sense of vulnerability, a loss of self-esteem, and anger. They experience a marked alteration in the quality of their life in all spheres, and the financial burden secondary to the illness is real and overwhelming. These issues can at times create instability in the emotional response to the illness and even result in discrete psychopathological processes, frequently of a depressive nature. Schizophrenic disorders and reactive psychoses are also seen, but adjustment disorders are the most common diagnosis, as is true of the general cancer population at this center.

In the psychiatric evaluation of AIDS patients, it is essential to consider organic mental syndromes that can resemble functional psychiatric illness. It is important to conduct a careful mental status examination to elicit the subtle cognitive changes that differentiate between neurologically impaired and depressed patients. Gross symptoms of organic mental disorder, such as disorientation, memory deficits, and visual hallucinations, may also occur.

Snider et al. (1) reviewed 50 patients with neurological complications, representing 31 percent of all AIDS cases seen at this center (see also Chapter 3).

The psychiatric interventions used in management of AIDS patients included brief psychotherapy, conjoint psychotherapy between a gay patient and his partner, and psychotropic medication (anxiolytics, major tranquilizers, and antidepressants). One patient required psychiatric hospitalization for bizarre behavior and a thought disorder. Psychotherapy was of a brief, supportive type; however, patients were followed from consultation through the course of their illness. The goals of psychotherapy included a facilitation of coping strategies, the development of support systems in more isolated patients, and the development of the ability to cope with the reemergence of an emotional distress similar to that of "coming out."

In some patients, the onset of AIDS caused them to reexperience the feelings and fantasies engendered at the time in their lives when they accepted themselves as homosexual. It was of therapeutic benefit in these cases to explore these reactions with the patient.

Psychotropic medications were used. Low-dose major tranquilizers (chlorpromazine equivalents of 50–200 mg per day) were given to patients who showed severe anxiety, organic mental syndromes with agitation, or a psychotic or acute schizophrenic episode.

An iatrogenic cause of depression in this population of patients should be mentioned. Our center sees a large number of KS patients who are frequently treated with human leukocyte interferon. The protocol calls for a daily injection of interferon for 21 to 60 days, followed by injections three times a week for an extended period of time. Within the first week, side effects are produced, which may include malaise, lethargy, loss of interest, hypersomnia, loss of appetite, hopelessness, and even suicidal thoughts.

The following case report summarizes the depressive sequelae that may be seen with this treatment. The patient was a white homosexual man who had had KS for seven months. Psychiatric consultation was requested to evaluate his depression and the risk of suicide. He had led an isolated lifestyle with no ongoing interpersonal ties and had a negative outlook on life. He found it difficult to trust people and had only rare, anonymous sexual contacts. His childhood had been spent in a nonsupportive family environment. When KS was first diagnosed, he procured drugs and alcohol with an intent to commit suicide.

The patient had been receiving daily injections of interferon for a week and had experienced shaking chills, depression, and physical debilitation. He was embarrassed by the KS lesions on his face, which he attempted to cover up with makeup, and he was concerned about becoming dependent on others. He admitted some suicidal thoughts but denied that he was about to attempt it; he was not considered a suicidal risk at the time. He appeared tired and depressed and exhibited hopelessness, a loss of self-esteem, and a concern that he was becoming a burden to the staff. He was not interested in psychotherapy. Desipramine was started at 50 mg at bedtime and was raised to 100 mg after three nights. He was referred to the "KS information group" at the center with the hope that improved socialization would develop. Ten days later he complained of feeling worse but did not want to discontinue the interferon, and he denied suicidal ideas. Desipramine was increased to 150 mg at bedtime. Four days later the patient was found to have killed himself at home.

Another case report illustrates the treatment of an individual with an organic brain syndrome. The patient was a 38-year-old homosexual actor who reported a wide range of substance abuse in the past. He was hospitalized for pneumonia, which was being treated with trimethoprim-sulfamethoxazole (Bactrim), when he developed nighttime agitation and visual hallucinations. There was no recent drug or alcohol abuse, and his blood gases were normal. On examination, he appeared cathectic and exhibited recent memory defects and intermittent confusion. He was given halodiperidol, 1 mg three times daily, and improvement was noted by the second day: he was less agitated and confused, and the hallucinations had remitted. The patient later died of respiratory collapse, and an autopsy revealed herpes simplex lesions in the brain.

The third case report shows the titration of antidepressants during the course of KS. The patient was a 47-year-old homosexual man who, as his facial KS lesions progressed, became anxious, depressed, and experienced unrelenting fearful thoughts and an appetite and sleep disturbance. He had undergone a brief course of psychotherapy in the past, but otherwise there was no psychiatric history in the patient or his family. The patient was successful in the fashion industry, had a close supportive male friend, and his lifetime sexual activity was limited to several monogamous relationships. On examination he was an anxious, agitated man who expressed hopelessness and despair and reported frequent, impulsive thoughts of suicide. Insomnia, poor appetite, and a lack of motivation were also present. He was given imipramine, and the dose was raised to 100 mg daily after 15 days. Symptoms did not improve, but he developed lightheadedness and a severe dry mouth. The dose was lowered to 50 mg, and then raised slowly through 75 mg to 100 mg daily; one week later improvement was noted in his mood. Although his facial disfiguration worsened, he responded with less anxiety and despair and began to take more interest in his care and to accept help from others.

Tricyclic antidepressants were given to patients who were diagnosed as having an adjustment disorder with depressed mood. They responded to low-dose (up to 100 mg per day) antidepressant therapy. An interesting and unexplained finding at our center is that, in general, cancer patients respond to antidepressants in lower doses than patients without cancer do.

Psychological and social interventions are an integral part of treatment, for without adequate coping strategies and environmental supports, patients are easily lost from follow-up care. In this context, many patients are referred to the Gay Men's Health Crisis in New York City, which provides a variety of important services to patients with AIDS.

Reference

1. Snider WD, Simpson DM, Nielsen S, et al: Neurological complications of acquired immune deficiency syndrome: analysis of 50 patients. Ann Neurol 14:403–418, 1983

7

Social and Support Groups for Patients with Acquired Immune Deficiency Syndrome

Stuart E. Nichols, M.D.

7

Social and Support Groups for Patients with Acquired Immune Deficiency Syndrome

The psychological adjustment of persons with AIDS and with the nonspecific AIDS-related syndrome is facilitated by social and support groups. Some of the advantages and pitfalls of each are presented here.

Because AIDS is so frequently fatal, the emotional reaction to it includes the responses to death and dying about which Kübler-Ross has written (1). However, because persons with AIDS are frequently estranged from their families, the support networks that usually ameliorate the psychologic reactions to dying may not be available to patients. A number of organizations (the Shanti Project, the AIDS/Kaposi Foundations, the Gay Men's Health Crisis, etc.) have attempted to provide the services normally expected from the family; these agencies are an invaluable resource for physicians treating AIDS patients (see also Chapter 10).

Two dangerous psychological reactions confront newly diagnosed patients: shock and denial (see Chapter 5 for additional discussion of these reactions). Thoughts of suicide may be among the first reactions to AIDS, and a psychiatric consultation is often warranted during the workup or at the time of diagnosis. Medication may be needed to ease the initial shock, and, unless a rapport is established early, it may be difficult to get the patient to cooperate with a psychiatrist later.

SOCIAL PROGRAMS

A support group is often too frightening an experience for a recently diagnosed patient, but an organized social program (group outings, theater parties, sports activities, etc.) may allow the individual to begin to interact with other persons with AIDS as it counteracts the tendency to isolation. These programs were devised, in part, to minimize the dangerous reaction of denial, which may jeopardize patients' health and deprive them of needed medical, psychological, and social support. The group should be structured so that it minimizes the illness and emphasizes the activity. The composition of social groups has been variable; successful programs have limited attendance to persons with AIDS, while others have included friends and family. Social programs are valuable for patients throughout the course of their illness. Denial tends to recur periodically in the course of the illness, and these programs assist persons during those periods until the time when they are able to deal with the full range of their emotions in the support group.

THE SUPPORT GROUP

In addition, adjustment to a support group may be facilitated by making it open-ended. This allows patients to attend periodically, each session exposing them to other patients and their individual reactions to the illness. Through this process many persons have overcome their resistance and have become ongoing members of the group.

One must be mindful of the disturbing effect of a newly formed group. Until a group has developed its own appropriate rules of conduct and style of operation, it is likely that the turbulence of the formation process may frighten new patients and reinforce their resistances. As mentioned in Chapter 4, some participants may have strong fears of intimacy that make it difficult for them to adjust to a group. Physicians who refer patients even to an established group should follow them carefully during the initial adjustment, exploring their reactions and helping them to understand and accept the feelings that may overwhelm them.

AIDS groups have been organized by hospital social workers, gay mental health professionals, and agencies that specialize in caring for the terminally ill. These groups are, in some cases, restricted by diagnosis (Kaposi's sarcoma only, Kaposi's sarcoma and opportunistic infections only, persons with nonspecific symptomatology, etc.). The support group described in this chapter is now conducted by persons who themselves have AIDS, using a structure modeled after Alcoholics Anonymous; nonpatients may attend the meetings once a month.

The perception of AIDS as a "homosexual disease" has been especially unfortunate for nongays who have developed this perception. Intravenous drug users are as diverse a group as homosexuals and, like gays, are stereotyped. They have not formed a community effort capable of providing peer support. Narcotics Anonymous groups have been helpful to some, especially those for whom abstinence from drugs is a personal goal. The gay community has provided most of the support services to this group, and through these exchanges each group has discovered some of its false preconceptions about the other.

Haitians seem to find it especially difficult to turn to the gay community for assistance, and it may be that they are the adult patient group with the least social and psychological support. (Children with AIDS, however, may have the most difficulty of all in obtaining appropriate supportive services because of the unfounded fear that they may be a danger to other children.) Since the outbreak of AIDS, any black with a foreign accent is likely to be regarded with considerable suspicion, and even healthy Haitians have been subjected to increased discrimination. Because of this, and the panicky fears of contagion, recent immigrants have sometimes been rejected by their own established community.

THE ADJUSTMENT PROCESS

The support group has followed what has been described as a rehabilitative approach—facilitating change through techniques similar to those used in alcoholism, drug addiction, and physical rehabilitation. The adjustment that many patients are capable of making in such a group is described below.

In the group, patients learn to take responsibility for their own reactions to AIDS. They help each other to identify any unreasonableness, ferreting out the magical, infantile, and superstitious thoughts which color their response. Self-pity and the foolhardy attempts to figure out why they got sick are discouraged. Hysteria is turned aside with reason and reassurance. Patients may be frightened, angry, sad, or in pain, but they learn that, while they must accept the conditions that AIDS imposes, they still have the ability to control their attitudes, make their own decisions, and manage their lives. They no longer see treatment as something done to them by doctors; persons with AIDS (as they prefer to be called rather than AIDS victims or even AIDS patients) become active participants in decisions about their care. Frequently they augment traditional care with keen attention to diet, adequate rest, exercise, relaxation, and the therapeutic techniques of holistic medicine such as macrobiotics, meditation, megavitamins, and positive imaging.

Concomitantly, patients scrutinize the quality of their lives, conducting a fearless examination for the sources of pain and pleasure. In this comprehensive review, they consider almost everything that touches their existence: health, drugs, and sex; companionship, affection, and intimacy; truth, courage, trust, and good will. They learn to dismiss the quick fix of instant pleasure and to appreciate the importance of deeper, more satisfying pleasures. Whatever makes life more satisfying must be pursued, whatever does not is rejected. Individuals are encouraged to be scrupulously honest. As a result, values and behavior can change rapidly. Many discover the strength to be the persons they had always wanted to be, and they create more satisfaction in their lives than they had thought possible.

In taking responsibility for the quality of one's life, there isn't one standard answer for everyone; each must decide what is best for him. For example, when sex is discussed there are two unavoidable considerations. Patients must protect themselves from a disease which could kill them in their immunocompromised state; in addition, they must limit sex to activities which will not endanger their partners. New patients often choose not to have sex at all as the simplest way to shoulder the responsibility. With time, many patients develop monogamous relationships or learn to avoid sexual activity in which body secretions are passed from one individual to another. In this regard, persons with AIDS have written and published their own recommendations for safe sex (2).

Finally, each patient makes a conscious decision to increase his sense of being alive. Patients encourage one another to live each day to the fullest extent possible. Persons who reach this stage of adjustment report that they feel more vibrant, spiritual, spontaneous, and content despite their pain. They had not imagined such a state of aliveness was possible before AIDS. They spend considerable time in helping others; their altruism varies from quiet personal support to community service.

This is a remarkable transformation: those who are facing death are serene. They have found a calmness in the midst of chaos; the healthy public remains frightened and panicky. Of course, this adjustment is not achieved by every patient, and even those who do are not able to maintain it all the time. Persons with AIDS talk of the "roller coaster ride" of the disease, a metaphor for the ups and downs of their physical and emotional states. Nevertheless, participation in a support group has given many of them the ability to face life as well as death. This experience might be of help to all of us in allaying our own fears and allowing us to embrace life more lovingly. Psychiatrists should benefit from familiarity with this remarkable phenomenon.

References

1. Kübler-Ross E: On Death and Dying. New York, Macmillan, 1969

2. Berkowitz R, Callen M: How to Have Sex in an Epidemic. Edited by Dworkin R. New York, News From The Front, 1983

SOCIAL RESPONSES

It should be obvious from the previous section that the effects of AIDS are being felt at all levels of society. In this section, the authors examine the effects of AIDS on society itself, to determine the role that psychiatry should play in facilitating a reasonable response to the illness. In Chapter 8, Dr. Nichols describes the overall social climate, especially the current views of sexuality, to provide us with an understanding of the dominant forces in society that have shaped the reaction to AIDS. These forces must be taken into account if the efforts to minimize AIDS-related suffering are to be effective. In Chapter 9, Dr. Ostrow describes the responses of the health care system to AIDS, providing us with examples of both positive and negative reactions to this major health emergency. Then, in Chapter 10, Dr. Tavares and Mr. López describe how the community that is most directly affected has reacted, giving us a picture of the diversity in the gay community, its development of an enviable support network, and the unique spirit of cooperation that has been created between it and the major community.

Psychiatrists must also contribute their expertise to the AIDS research now getting underway. In Chapter 11, Dr. Michael Ross, an Australian psychiatrist and venereologist, discusses the newly emerging field of psychovenereology and its potential contributions to the understanding of the epidemic. His transcultural studies of the psychological, social, and political correlates of homosexual behavior are an example of the needed psychiatric research. In Chapter 12, Dr. Harold Alan Pincus, Special Assistant to the Director of the National Institute of Mental Health and head of the Ad Hoc NIMH Committee on AIDS, summarizes the current agenda for research into the mental health aspects of this unprecedented medical mystery.

In the epilogue that follows, Dr. James Krajeski gives an overview of the opportunities which AIDS presents to the psychiatric profession. He points out how, even at this early stage of incomplete understanding, psychiatry can help to heal the societal wounds produced by AIDS and provides us with positive goals for the future.

8

The Social Climate When the Acquired Immune Deficiency Syndrome Developed

Stuart E. Nichols, M.D.

8

The Social Climate When the Acquired Immune Deficiency Syndrome Developed

The acquired immune deficiency syndrome (AIDS) is a mysterious new disease that is difficult to diagnose, incurable, and devastating. Perhaps its most mysterious characteristic has been its predilection for already stigmatized subgroups within our society.

AIDS can now be traced back to 1979. Although it has always been found most frequently among male homosexuals, the percentages of cases in each of the risk groups (gay men, intravenous drug users, Haitians, and hemophiliacs) has remained amazingly constant. Therefore, AIDS has posed little threat to the general population; it is not spread casually from person to person. Nevertheless, many people continue to experience an excessive fear of exposure to it. Could it be that the popular perception of AIDS as a "gay disease" is causing much of the hysteria that surrounds the illness?

It seems as if the traditional dread of homosexuality has become part of the irrational reaction to AIDS. Do some persons feel themselves to be already infected with unacceptable desire, which, if exposed, would destroy them? Or is the fear that of unrestrained sexuality, which some people associate with homosexuality? Our puritan heritage proclaims sex to be dirty and sinful; unrestrained sexual activity, even masturbation, invites divine retribution. The scare produced by genital herpes may be an indication that this fear of retribution still exists in many persons, often on an unconscious level. If so, one would expect an even stronger reaction to AIDS, which is associated in the public mind with unrestrained homosexuality.

The psychiatric implications of an illness such as AIDS cannot be understood apart from the milieu in which it is found. No brief discussion can enumerate all the influences that have affected the reaction to AIDS; such a presentation is beyond the scope, length, and expertise of this monograph. In the hope of facilitating a reasonable perspective toward this syndrome, however, this chapter will point out certain psychosocial forces that have, at least in part, shaped society's reaction to AIDS.

In ancient times a raging epidemic was often thought to be the punishment from an offended god. In the twentieth century, some people still regard a few diseases in this magical way, chief among them are cancer and venereal disease. Until recently "VD" was an uncontrollable threat to mankind. Sexually transmitted diseases were said to have decimated civilizations and detoured the course of history. To some people such devastation testified to the seriousness of sexual transgression. The possibility that fleeting pleasure could be followed by never-ending retribution made sex more tempting as forbidden fruit, yet also infinitely more terrifying. Stringent rules regarding proper masculine, feminine, and sexual behavior were imposed by human society in an attempt to control lustful nature.

In addition, Judeo-Christian patriarchal tradition had ensured the dominance of men by regarding women as property; women had no inheritance rights, no vote, and even no control over their own bodies. "Normal" women were also denied the right to sexual appetite and pleasure.

One result of society's perceived need to limit sexuality was the discouragement of a scientific study of the subject. Although it was occasionally investigated, more frequently in Europe than in America, these studies had little impact on popular thinking prior to Freud. Later, when Kinsey published his landmark *Sexual Behavior in the Human Male*, he was attacked by the president of Princeton who compared it to "toilet wall inscriptions," and the book prompted a professor at Columbia University to call "for a law against doing research exclusively with sex" (1). With such a strong taboo, it is not surprising that our concepts of sexuality at the time were flawed.

Kinsey's research was greeted with astonishment and jeers, but it encouraged people to begin to talk and think differently about sex. Even so, it was not until the late 1960s that his work was truly accepted. The countercultural youth of that day were not alarmed by the rather widespread homosexual activity in our society; many young people had experimented with it. They also seemed to accept with ease the concept of a continuum between heterosexuality and homosexuality, and the idea that they could be attracted to either gender at different times.

The 1960s were a decade of social revolution. At the time American youth perceived the nation to be hypocritical in conducting itself in ways at variance with its supposed moral standards. Kenneth Boulding has described the process of social change as occurring in two phases: an educational movement that offers society new concepts, followed by a protest movement, or rebellion, that forces it to alter the way it acts. Boulding has described the difference between the two as follows:

> A protest movement needs to be shrill, obstreperous, undignified, and careless of the existing legitimacy which it is seeking to destroy in the interest of a new pattern which is waiting to emerge. Educational movements have to be low-keyed, respectful of existing legitimacies, tying into them whenever possible, and chary of arousing counterprotest. . . .When the movement for protest arrives, however, the educational institution is often pushed aside, and perhaps properly so, as inappropriate in the circumstances (2).

The protest movements of the 1960s produced enormous change in the nation. Blacks, women, and gay people wrested freedoms for themselves that had been undreamed of a generation before, and they assumed new roles in the social, economic, and political spheres. The sexual revolution was made possible, in part, by the liberation movements, by the development of powerful and readily available antibiotics and effective birth control, and by the legalization of abortion. Sex was no longer a restricted, procreative act where pleasure was secondary; it was now increasingly accepted as a normal and natural experience of erotic fulfillment for everyone. It became easily available to many persons, seemingly with no drawbacks. The stigma of venereal disease was removed; sexually transmitted diseases (STDs) were considered no more distressing than a headache and no more embarrassing. The spiraling rates of STDs in the 1970s attested to the changed sexual practices (3).

Besides the breaking of sexual taboos, society experienced other fundamental and sweeping changes. Divorce was no longer regarded as stigmatizing and became increasingly more prevalent. The traditional family was replaced in many cases by innovations in ways of relating to lovers and raising children. Parents were less able to control the education of their children. Books could still be banned from school libraries, but many youngsters were now getting much of their knowledge from television; the pictures of people, places, and behavior they saw there expanded the children's perspective, oftentimes in a manner objectionable to parents.

The Great Society's coinciding with the Vietnam conflict fostered disillusionment with a government and society that had promised more than it could deliver; this lack of faith reached its apogee with Watergate. The multiplication of "entitlement programs" whetted the appetites and the expectations of a segment of the population. After Vietnam, drugs were no longer a big-city phenomenon; across the country persons were using drugs either as recreation or out of desperation. Advances in transportation had made the world shrink. The death of nationalism and the invalidation of isolationism was replaced by a new global awareness.

It is axiomatic that change created by revolution breeds unrest and counterrevolution. By the end of the 1970s, a deep division existed in the country, a line drawn roughly between youth and their elders. Youth extolled the advanced virtues of the new wave; traditionalists decried what they called the loss of principle in our behavior. For them, the cold war threat of outside attack had been pushed aside by the fear of internal subversion. Some persons confused preservation of the status quo with stability. The nation was poised for change.

At this time, the outbreaks of Legionnaires' disease and toxic-shock syndrome gave the nation a brief scare; some people associated toxic-shock syndrome with the new sexuality. Not surprisingly, with the outbreak of an STD that modern medicine could not cure—recrudescent, recurring genital herpes—the country was panic-stricken. But finally, with AIDS, the country reacted with frank hysteria. Human society rediscovered its dread of uncontrollable disease, and the conservative forces in our society had a cause around which to rally.

Thus, the reactions to AIDS were shaped by the pull of the social tides of revolution and reaction. The shattering of many of society's fundamental tenets and taboos in the preceding two decades gave these forces exceptional strength at that time.

A reexamination of our concepts of human sexuality may help us to deal with AIDS more rationally. Kinsey's research showed us a possible reason why sexual studies had been shunned previously: he found much more homosexual experience in the society than it acknowledged. These results have been verified by subsequent research at the Institute for Sexual Research at Indiana University, which recently documented homosexual fantasy in every individual tested (4). Therefore, the investigation of sexuality threatened to reveal a secret that the society had struggled to conceal; more importantly, it threatened to uncover the dreaded, stigmatizing trait in many individuals. This may explain much of our nervousness about sexuality. Even the perception of "safety" and the sexual excesses that followed the sexual revolution may represent, in part, a reaction formation to this anxiety. In any case, with AIDS the sense of danger resurfaced more vigorously than before. When panic is experienced by persons not at risk, it may be derived from the old fear of exposure—the fear of discovering homosexual feeling, not of contact with the putative AIDS agent.

Insight into the society's sexual anxiety is important beyond the understanding of AIDS. Psychiatrists must also understand that the impossible attempt to protect ourselves from our own sexual natures has dire consequences. Since the defense against our own homoerotic feeling requires that homosexuals be regarded as different, they are likely to be seen as inferior or even less human in some essential way. In troubled times they become ready targets for scapegoating.

With AIDS, scapegoating is encountered on a societal level as well as in individual care. For example, the early inadequate funding of research may betray the popular perception that gay people are different: AIDS is "their" problem, not "ours." The lapses in confidentiality that have occurred may reveal an attitude that "they" are less valuable than "regular" people. The attempt to deny all gay persons the ability to donate blood may show the prejudicial assumption that "they are all alike."

However, if human sexuality is thought of as being a continuum between heterosexuality and homosexuality in everyone, many of these problems would be minimized or eliminated. The sense of a basic difference between gay and nongay people would be removed, as would the imaginary danger now attached to the recognition of one's intrinsic homoerotic feeling. With such a conceptualization, psychiatrists could avoid the risky business of judging sexual normalcy; sexual behavior would be interpreted as the resultant interplay of social, psychodynamic, and biologic factors. This, indeed, is the point of view that psychiatry has taken in recent years, and this approach should be reinforced by the AIDS epidemic, which forces every physician to become more familiar with homosexuality. Nevertheless, there continues to be a need for basic research into the nature of human sexuality, investigations that are carefully constructed and carried out, reproducible, and scientific.

AIDS affords the nation many opportunities to expand knowledge; the insights gained here will guide the sexual practices of the post-AIDS era. It was learned, in the sexual revolution, that there are myriad forms of healthy adult sexuality. AIDS should strengthen the country's emerging concept that most homosexuals are competent, mature individuals. If America meets the challenges of AIDS, responding appropriately to its medical, psychological, and social crises, true social progress will result.

References

1. Tripp CA: The Homosexual Matrix. New York, McGraw-Hill, 1975, p 219

2. Boulding KE: Towards a theory of protest, in The Age of Protest. Edited by Anderson W. Pacific Palisades, California, Goodyear Publishing Co, 1969, p viii

3. Ostrow DG, Altman NL: Sexually transmitted disease and homosexuality. Sex Trans Dis 10: 208–215, 1983

4. Bell A, Weinberg MS, Hammersmith SK: Sexual Preference: Its Development in Men and Women. Bloomington, Ind, Indiana University Press, 1981

9

Medical Responses to Acquired Immune Deficiency Syndrome

David G. Ostrow, M.D., Ph.D.

9

Medical Responses to Acquired Immune Deficiency Syndrome

The new and deadly disease, acquired immune deficiency syndrome (AIDS), has had tremendous psychological effects on persons at risk, their communities, health care personnel, and the general population. This chapter will concentrate on examples of response which are understandable from the nature of the disease itself. By doing so, we can develop an understanding of why the AIDS phenomenon has had such profound effects and use this understanding to devise rational responses to it and develop effective ways of calming the public through education. Health providers must play a leadership role in handling AIDS and its protean implications. Some of the examples given illustrate inadequate responses or the drastic and sudden changes that AIDS can produce at all levels of society.

We begin by looking at the working definition of AIDS, as established by the Centers for Disease Control (CDC) over two years ago and which has remained essentially unchanged: "A life-threatening, unusual malignancy (such as Kaposi's sarcoma) in a person less than 60 years old, and/or a life-threatening opportunistic infection indicative of severe cellular immune deficiency in the absence of any known cause of immunosuppression." That definition makes AIDS a diagnosis of exclusion, as we must rule out any known causes of immunosuppression in patients before we can say that they have AIDS. This results in an extended period of diagnostic work-up, waiting, and uncertainty on the part of both the patient and the health care personnel. This is the first major factor coloring our responses to AIDS, namely the uncertainty associated with the disease.

The next problem is that the disease is usually fatal. The disease was uniformly fatal when first observed and continues to lead inexorably to death in the majority of patients, a situation which produces a tremendous sense of frustration in patients, health care workers, and the communities at risk. This frustration occurs because no matter what is done, no matter how diligent the medical response, the chance of survival is still quite low.

Third, the etiology is unknown, although the putative transmissible agent has now been identified. The definition of AIDS requires "no known cause of immunosuppression." Much research continues into the cause(s) of the immunosuppression underlying AIDS. Meanwhile, the lack of detailed knowledge about its etiology, the lack of knowledge about its cure, and the lack of knowledge about the ultimate numbers of patients who will suffer from this disease create fear. So we have three major characteristics of the AIDS phenomenon, namely uncertainty, frustration, and fear, emotions which cannot help but add up to hysteria and irrational reactions of society at large. This panic is even stronger in the patients themselves and in persons in direct contact with them.

The term "risk group" or "being at risk for AIDS" are themselves a major problem. It seems that a person diagnosed as having AIDS is classified in a social sense as well. There are few diseases that carry with them stigmas of such magnitude, and no disease before AIDS picked out its victims so selectively from such a broad list of socially stigmatized groups. A fourth aspect of AIDS, which certainly flavors medical response, is the stigma with which most of the groups at risk were regarded even before the disease. Perhaps an even more intense reaction occurs in persons with what may be precursor or prodromol states. We know that these must exist, but we are far from defining them clearly. We do know the nonspecific symptoms that indicate that some kind of problem might be brewing in patients. These often go undiagnosed, or are given the names of "lymphadenopathy syndrome," "pre-AIDS," or "AIDS-related complex." Many more people have one or more of these prodromal symptoms than have AIDS, and the prodromal symptoms, in themselves, lead to more uncertainty, frustration, and fear. Even healthy members of the risk groups may walk daily tightropes as to whether they are going to develop AIDS. They may feel guilty about behavior which has put them at risk in the past; they do not know if the change in behavior instituted on account of AIDS is really going to help them, since they could be already incubating a disease with a two-year or longer latency period. In addition, each risk group has its own special anxiety to contend with. Gay men have been blamed for the "gay plague," and addicts and hemophiliacs see the disease as yet another devastating complication to their ways of life. Finally there is the Haitian group: persons who entered the United States since 1979 rather than longstanding Haitian residents of the United States. The Haitian group illustrates the role of politics and stigma in the medical response to AIDS. Some researchers feel that by designating Haitians as a risk group we are causing further discrimination against a group already disadvantaged and highly discriminated against. The fact remains, however, that even after removing from the Haitian entrant group the known intravenous drug abusers and persons admitting to homosexual activity, there is still a considerable percentage of patients who are unexplained except for their membership in this group. We have to ask ourselves whether social problems like those encountered by recent Haitian entrants to the United States should lead to changes in our epidemiological classification. Does the attempt to reduce social stigma justify the scientific confusion which this type of action would produce? A positive consequence of debate on this issue has been the recognition that detailed understanding of the culture and society of Haitians living both in the United States and Haiti is an important and necessary part of our understanding of the causes of AIDS.

EFFECTS OF AIDS ON THE MEDICAL PROFESSION

Health care workers are themselves a potential AIDS risk group. Most health care workers in the United States have not yet had to deal directly with AIDS patients nor have to confront their own reactions to it. Working closely with an AIDS patient is a very sobering experience. When you have to tell someone that he has AIDS, and both you and he know that he is likely to die and that little or nothing can be done to help him, the sadness, depression, and isolation can be overwhelming. There is very little in the training of medical professionals that prepares them to handle such an experience. Added to it are the fears that we may have of being already contaminated or fears of becoming infected through working with AIDS patients, and we can begin to understand, if not excuse, some of the reactions to AIDS patients by some members of the health care professions. These include doctors and nurses who would not attend to AIDS patients, pregnant nurses who ask to be transferred off wards with AIDS patients, and doctors who avoid touching persons from AIDS risk groups.

We live in a time of increasing specialization, compartmentalization, and the resultant social isolation among various parts of the health care system. The medical profession, which has long had a tradition of overcoming social barriers and of being proud of the hands-on relationship between the clinician and the patient is now, in some instances, more interested in being sure that there is some kind of impervious barrier between us and the patient. This adds to our already increasing reliance on laboratory tests, microbiological isolations, and viral serologies instead of the one-to-one clinical interaction that we were taught in school, an interaction that may have been a major inducement for some to enter the medical profession.

Then we must consider the families and intimate contacts of AIDS patients. Such persons worry about the extent to which their relationships may have exposed them to this deadly disease. How can they continue to lead a normal life and at the same time have a close or intimate relationship with a person with AIDS? The household and intimate contacts of health care professionals caring for AIDS patients are known to have similar worries.

Thus we have come from the anxiety produced by the uncertainty, frustration, and fear—let's add ignorance—attached to AIDS; to hysterical, emotional, and sometimes irrational reactions to that anxiety; and to further anxieties produced by our responses to AIDS. Therefore, AIDS has created a vicious circle of psychological symptoms leading to specific responses, which in turn cause further psychological responses. How can we deal with this to minimize or, if possible, reverse the physical and psychological damage that has been done?

Responding to the Challenges of AIDS with Accurate Medical Information

First of all, we must deal with information that is based on fact. Local health departments and the CDC's AIDS Task Force make regular reports of confirmed AIDS cases in each major U.S. city, which is then further broken down by group characteristics, specific diagnoses, outcome, and various demographic factors. In Chicago, this information is collected on an ongoing basis and is disseminated each month by the Office of AIDS Activity of the Chicago Department of Health. That office was created, in part, to deal with the need for accurate facts to counter the various rumors that have circulated as the result of AIDS. Dr. Aaron Josephson, of the Mid-America Red Cross, has repeatedly appeared on television to assure viewers that AIDS cannot be contracted by giving blood. It is not an optimal use of our time to shoot down rumors of this type, but it is necessary to do all that we can to supplant rumor with fact. It takes a coordinated effort on the part of all the involved individuals, groups, and agencies to resolve, through education, the hysteria created by AIDS. That is why health departments in many U.S. cities are setting up offices or bureaus of AIDS activity to provide coordination, staff support, and educational materials to local community efforts.

Dealing with the news media—newspapers, magazines, radio, and television—is itself a very difficult and critical activity. Most of the American public now receives the majority of its medical information through these media. Combine the desire—indeed, the responsibility—of members of the news media to know as much as possible about AIDS with our relative ignorance about the disease, and again one can begin to understand aspects of the media's response to AIDS. An example of media hysteria occurred in the summer of 1983 when, immediately after a Saturday evening television news announcement of a possible transfusion-related AIDS case, I was besieged by reporters asking me about the case. I received a total of 142 media contacts related to that episode. The avalanche of media interest in AIDS is an awesome social phenomenon. At its roots are the same elements of fear, uncertainty, and frustration which underlie the general population's responses to AIDS. However, media hype leads to increased general concern, which, in turn, leads to increased media attention. On the positive side, we are witnessing an increasing sophistication on the part of certain media and segments of their audiences; hospital public relations personnel and the media are giving out more complicated medical information, which is often more understandable and difficult to distort.

No area of medical information is more sensitive at this time than the question of blood-borne transmission of AIDS. The "evidence" for blood transmission rests on about 30 cases in which no other risk factors have been identified. None of the donors has developed AIDS except in a handful of those cases, but a donor has been identified, in most cases, who either belongs to one of the risk groups or has some degree of altered cellular immunity. No smoking gun by any means, but the medical and social consequences are considerable.

Public hysteria has led to the call for a halt to blood donation by all members of the various risk groups, through voluntary means. This has produced, and continues to produce, a strong reaction. The suggestion that all members of a risk group may be unsuitable as blood donors automatically leads to measures to exclude them and segregate their blood on a categorical rather than medical basis. Worse, these actions may lead to further stigmatization of that group as having "bad blood," inspiring scapegoating, anger, and even reprisals. Further, such prohibitions are ultimately unenforceable. For example, closeted homosexuals might be tempted to donate blood to "prove" their heterosexuality. Thus, the need to protect blood recipients has clashed with the responsibility to not malign and stigmatize entire groups of individuals.

An uneasy compromise has been reached which calls for members of risk groups to refrain voluntarily from donating blood if they, on an individual basis, have any of the characteristics which would place them at high risk for exposure to AIDS. In particular, homosexual men with multiple sexual partners, with a known exposure to an AIDS patient, or with any of the prodromal symptoms were asked to withdraw from the donor pool. The debate on the role of blood transfusions in AIDS continues. Meanwhile, we are forced to ask ourselves just how far the health care system should go in its responsibility to protect an individual, when that action might infringe on the civil liberties and reputation of a whole group of individuals. This type of question cannot be easily answered and is an example of one of the basic ethical questions which AIDS raises and which must be addressed by both the medical profession and society at large.

Another problem occurs when members of the health care profession become unduly anxious about being contaminated by an agent(s) which may cause AIDS. The CDC has published guidelines on contagion control for AIDS. They call basically for the same precautions as with hepatitis B virus and other blood-borne viruses. It is a sociological observation to note that the tremendous effects the AIDS guidelines produced indicate how little we followed them in the past and are only now rushing to catch-up in this new and often fatal disease. Nevertheless, the guidelines have been interpreted in various ways. One major hospital in Chicago originally asked physicians to determine the sexual preference of each new patient. Male patients determined to be homosexual had their charts labeled "PVA" for potential viral agent. Thereafter, blood and other lab specimens from them were handled according to the recommendations for viral-contaminated materials. If the patient was hospitalized, hepatitis precautions were taken. This may have seemed like a reasoned, intelligent response to AIDS, but was it? In the first place, it was based on a physician's assessment of their patients' sexual orientation. Few physicians actually ask about sexual orientation but assume that they know what it is from their patient's behavior or marital status. With AIDS, the medical profession may finally realize that sexual orientation and a specific history of sexual practices are an important component of the medical evaluation of any sexually active patient. In addition, by following the CDC guidelines, medical centers can avoid inappropriate contagion control measures with AIDS patients.

Those of us who were involved in the establishment of sexually transmitted disease (STD) clinics serving the gay community have felt that such clinics would be unnecessary if mainstream medicine took an interest in these problems, incorporated them into the medical educational system, and handled them in a confidential and nonjudgmental way. Instead, with AIDS, we now see the development of a separate way of handling homosexual men within mainstream institutions. This is a major sociological change in the way medical care is delivered. Are we moving towards the segregation of gay patients within our medical systems, much the same way that we have segregated chronic mental patients?

There are already cases of AIDS among health care workers who belong to a risk group, and there will inevitably be cases of AIDS among health care workers with no known risk factor other than taking care of AIDS patients. Furthermore, we have to look at the potential economic impact of AIDS on the practice of medicine. If and when we know the full spectrum of AIDS diseases, and whether or not there are carrier states with healthy individuals capable of transmitting the disease to others, we may have formidable questions to deal with. In some quarters questions are even now being raised about homosexual and Haitian health care professionals merely because of their categorical membership in an AIDS risk group, but to date, there haven't been clear-cut examples of prejudicial action toward them. The imminent, widespread introduction of serological tests for a putative AIDS etiologic agent, HTLV III or LAV (which may be the same virus), before we have sufficient information regarding its transmissibility and the clinical consequences of infection, will undoubtedly lead to even more serious ethical problems.

In regard to the social and occupational behaviors of AIDS patients themselves, there is a problem that increases as time goes on and as persons with AIDS survive for one, two, and three years or more. This group, "People with AIDS," proclaim that they are active, contributing members of society and are not to be seen as victims of the disease or as lepers. Should they be allowed to work in areas where there may be potential for transmission of AIDS? Should they remain sexually active, and, if so, in what ways? How far should the treating physician go in dissuading an AIDS patient from engaging in practices which are potentially dangerous to both the patient and his contacts? Again we are confronted with the conflict between the rights of persons with AIDS, individuals with needs and concerns similar to those of others, and the role of medicine to protect patients and society. This is a very basic question that now confronts us as the result of AIDS. It will be several years before we fully understand the epidemiologic consequences of infection with HTLV III, LAV, and perhaps other putative AIDS etiologic agents. In the meantime, medicine will have to deal with uncertainties and ambiguities which will test our reasonableness and compassion.

MEDICAL RESPONSES TO AIDS: THE FUTURE

Since AIDS is a new disease, it is difficult to predict its long-term social and medical effects. We can, however, look at the effects of prior epidemics of fatal diseases; obvious examples are the medical response to leprosy, syphilis, cholera, and bubonic plague. Each of these diseases produced frustration, fear, and uncertainty in individuals, the health care professions, and government. Included in the medical response to these diseases were attempts at scapegoating specific social groups and then isolating them from the larger society to avoid contamination.

In subtle but undeniable ways, AIDS is producing similar responses. Within the medical profession there is a tendency to assume that there are social, behavioral, or geographic "origins" of

AIDS which are not based on scientific fact. Recent moves to bar the use of blood from entire metropolitan areas by blood product manufacturers are obvious examples of this type of response. Just as important are the insidious changes in how we treat patients depending on their social and economic backgrounds. Each step towards the segregation of health care facilities for homosexual, Haitian, or intravenous drug–using patients must be looked at carefully, and the long-term consequences of isolation and stigmatization must be weighed against the sometimes arguable benefits. Our response to AIDS is both a tremendous medical and social challenge, producing major changes in how we practice medicine, how we live our lives, and how we think about issues of individual freedom and social responsibility *all at the same time*. If we think about these changes in an orderly way, and talk about them among ourselves and with our families, patients, and friends, then these changes have tremendous promise for creating social progress. If we do not do so but respond with hysteria, fear, ignorance, uncertainty, and prejudice, the AIDS tragedy will be magnified many times over, and the losses in terms of human dignity, understanding, and kindness will be devastating. As members of the healing professions, we must redouble our efforts to ensure that we contribute towards positive social responses to AIDS.

10

Response of the Gay Community to Acquired Immune Deficiency Syndrome

Rafael Tavares, M.D.
Diego J. López, C.S.W.

10

Response of the Gay Community to Acquired Immune Deficiency Syndrome

In 1980, a small group of gay men in New York City began to meet to discuss the recent deaths of some of their close friends. Out of these meetings the Gay Men's Health Crisis (GMHC) was founded to respond to the mysterious health threat. Almost simultaneously, throughout the nation in areas affected by the acquired immune deficiency syndrome (AIDS), agencies began to address the medical and psychosocial problems it creates—established organizations (like the Shanti Project in San Francisco, the Gay and Lesbian Community Services Center in Los Angeles, the Howard Brown Memorial Clinic in Chicago, and the Whitman-Walker Clinic in Washington, D.C.) as well as new agencies (such as the AIDS/Kaposi Foundation in several major cities).

The services that these organizations offer have played an essential role in the care of AIDS patients and persons close to them. Interested readers can obtain information about the services that may be available in their communities through the AIDS Hotline which is maintained by the National Gay Task Force: (800) 221-7044. Most of these programs are conducted by gay mental health professionals, but they offer services to any person who has or who is concerned about AIDS.

The psychosocial needs of persons with AIDS identified by these agencies include emotional support to counteract feelings of isolation and helplessness; psychological intervention to address issues such as guilt, loss of control, denial, anger, depression, anxiety, and death and dying; and specific social services to help patients cope with legal, financial, social, and medical issues and the potentially overwhelming losses of income, employment, housing, independence, and autonomy.

A variety of innovative programs have been developed to meet these needs; those offered by GMHC illustrate one system of service delivery:

Crisis Intervention Counseling. A counselor establishes contact with a newly diagnosed patient to offer immediate emotional and psychological support, which continues as long as necessary, guides the patient through the often confusing procedures of the medical system, and follows up with a needs assessment of psychological and social services to which the patient is directed. The counselor keeps written records of all contact with the patient and other persons involved in the patient's care and maintains regular contact after the crisis phase of adjustment to AIDS to ensure that the patient is continuing to receive support services.

AIDS Therapy Groups. These groups are appropriate for persons with various manifestations of the disease who are able to confront the social, emotional, and behavioral consequences of AIDS.

Care Partners' Groups. These groups serve lovers, spouses, and friends of patients.

Parents' Support Groups. This program assists parents to express and deal with their own feelings as their children struggle with the illness.

Social Activities. Recreation groups help patients to counter the tendency to isolation and to work through their denial of the illness. They also facilitate a relaxed atmosphere between patients and nonpatients.

Buddy Support System. The patient's buddy helps in a limited capacity, such as with light housework, shopping, phone calls, care for a pet when the patient is hospitalized, etc.

Religious and Spiritual Counseling. Pastoral counselors are available to patients who request this service; the involved clergy have special instruction concerning AIDS.

Financial Advocacy Program. This program assists patients with third-party reimbursement and the governmental programs for financial aid.

Psychiatric Consultation. This is available for persons who experience psychiatric difficulties as a result of the illness. Individual psychotherapy is available on a limited basis for persons who are inappropriate for or who do not desire group therapy.

"Worried Well" Groups. These groups serve individuals who do not have AIDS but experience anxiety about it.

Much of the early factual information about AIDS was reported in the gay press at a time when the general media was either ignoring or sensationalizing the problem. Bobby Campbell, R.N., in San Francisco's *Sentinel*, Nathan Fain in the national newspaper *The Advocate*, and James D'Eramo and Lawrence Mass, M.D., in New York's *Native* wrote about the epidemic to a concerned readership.

The first national medical symposium to feature AIDS was held by the Bay Area Physicians for Human Rights in June 1981 and has been repeated annually. At the 1981 meeting a national gay medical organization was formed, the American Association of Physicians for Human Rights (AAPHR), which now has chapters throughout North America. AAPHR and many of its local affiliates have played important roles in assisting the health establishment to address the medical problems of AIDS in a reasonable manner. They have also served the gay community by advising it about altering sexual activity to reduce the risk for AIDS.

In August 1982, a gay leadership conference was held in Dallas. The National Gay Health Education Foundation (NGHEF) sponsored a special section of that meeting for individuals and agencies working with AIDS. A national AIDS network held its first official meeting in June 1983 in Denver and formed the Federation of AIDS Related Organization. Patients contributed to the delibera tions at this meeting and established their own organization, Persons with AIDS. In June 1984, the First International Gay and Lesbian Health Conference was held in New York City, again sponsored by NGHEF.

The story of the gay community response involves more than the work of concerned organizations; the illness has had a marked personal impact on individuals and a way of life. AIDS has caused a painful process of self-examination and mourning—not just for persons with AIDS but for their friends and lovers as well. The response of many individuals has been one of concern, first for themselves, but it has also allowed them to reach out and comfort others. The gay community has become the family that many of the affected individuals do not have—a living, loving, caring, sorrowing gay family. The development of this cohesive support network has also changed the focus of the gay community. AIDS was discovered just 12 years after the Stonewall riots marked the beginning of an open gay community, not a very long time for community development before it must tackle a crisis of this magnitude. Fortunately the community has grown to meet the challenges of AIDS.

One of the first changes involved medical care. Prior to AIDS there was good reason for a gay patient to hide his sexual orientation. By so doing he did not offend treatment personnel and avoided stigmatization. AIDS make concealment impossible, and many patients were subjected to horrible treatment, especially in the initial hysteria that greeted the disease. Persons with AIDS and some brave gay health care professionals have worked to ensure appropriate and dignified care for patients.

To nongay persons this may seem to be a fundamental right, but it was not until the AIDS crisis that the gay community began to realize that it had a right to be honest, open, and reasonable care, and that is was the obligation of medical administrators and public health officials to see that such care was given. Thus, the gay community and the medical establishment began to interact for the first time. From the onset of the illness, the Centers for Disease Control (CDC) had sought out the thinking of the gay community on AIDS. The leading institution of the gay community, the National Gay Task Force (NGTF), has become increasingly involved with the governmental response to AIDS beginning with the discovery of possible transfusion transmission of the illness in the summer of 1982. Virginia Apuzzo, director of NGTF, has been invaluable in establishing a working relationship between the two communities. Credit also goes to Roger Enlow and Bruce Voeller, who represented NGTF in discussions of blood-banking policy, and David Sencer, head of the Health Department in New York City, who personally invited gay participation in planning the response to AIDS and created the innovative Office for Lesbian and Gay Health Concerns within his department. In many cities across the country, AIDS has led to closer working relationships between local public health agencies and the gay community.

In summary, the gay community can take pride in its response to AIDS. It has met the crisis in supportive care for persons with AIDS and has offered its services to all affected individuals. It has helped to establish communication with important health care and governmental institutions, which has led to close and mutually beneficial working relationships. It has learned of the dangers of being isolated and alienated from the mainstream of society and recognized the vital interdependence of all groups in our society. Despite its uneasiness with the concept of gay liberation, the world should be thankful that an open and organized community was in existence when AIDS was discovered. How much suffering would have been added to this terrible disease if there was no gay community response? How much needless prejudice might have been unleashed had not gay people served as the nation's conscience in this epidemic?

11

Psychovenereology and Acquired Immune Deficiency Syndrome

Michael W. Ross, B.S. Med., Ph.D.

11

Psychovenereology and Acquired Immune Deficiency Syndrome

Psychovenereological considerations in acquired immune deficiency syndrome (AIDS) are of necessity limited to those cases in which AIDS is sexually transmitted. Such cases usually involve male homosexuals: Pinching et al. (1) note that with AIDS, homosexuals remain of central importance, comprising some 75 percent of all cases and having no underlying disorder apart from their propensity for contracting sexually transmitted diseases. Cases in which transmission occurs through intravenous drug therapy or abuse, or by way of blood or blood products, cannot be considered to be sexually transmitted: this is underscored by recent investigations by the World Health Organization in central Africa, in which about 40 percent of AIDS cases were women, and a significant proportion of these virgins. This chapter therefore focuses on male homosexuals and psychological factors involved in AIDS transmission.

There are two factors which in theory may be associated with infection with a sexually transmitted disease: the most obvious of these is partner numbers, where an increase in partners will increase the probability of sexually transmitted disease. The second is anonymity of partner, which appears to be to some degree independent of partner numbers. It is possible that the dynamic involved in anonymity of partner is related not to partner numbers as such but to the meeting of other individuals who themselves are more likely to have had multiple partners. An alternative explanation could be that those individuals who seek anonymous sex have lower resistance to infection, via reduced immune competence. This latter explanation suggests that psychological factors which may lower immune competence (Ader [2] has demonstrated that immune function may be conditioned) are also involved in preference for anonymous sex; this is, however, speculative and not based upon empirical findings.

The relationship between number of partners and number of infections is, however, unclear. Jaffe et al. (3) found highly significant associations between anonymous sex, syphilis infection, and number of partners. On the other hand, my own data on homosexual men in Sweden, Australia, Finland, and the Republic of Ireland found no significant associations between number of partners and frequency of infections with sexually transmitted disease except in the Irish sample. However, Jaffe et al. were looking at a sample of homosexual men with AIDS and matched controls who reported partner numbers per year of 61 and 27, respectively, as contrasted with my data, which showed a range from 39.6 (Sweden) to 20 per year (Finland) (4). It may be that there is a point beyond which there is an association between partner numbers, numbers of infections, and anonymity of sex. On the other hand, the sample described by Jaffe et al. came from AIDS patients and clinic attendees, whereas my sample was from the homosexual communities of the four countries studied, and unrelated to clinic attendance. It is most likely that samples consisting of those attending clinics or patients with sexually transmitted diseases constitute a biased group who are most likely to become infected, and thus findings cannot be generalized too readily to other homosexual men.

What are the findings with regard to the psychovenereology of partner numbers and number of infections? Looking at over 600 sexually active homosexual men in Sweden, Australia, Finland, and Ireland, I found that the best predictors of the number of times individuals had been infected with a sexually transmitted disease was *not* number of partners, but a set of psychological variables (5,

6). Surprisingly, while these variables could predict between 19 percent and 42 percent of the variance attributed to number of infections, six variables were common across countries. These were sex role as measured by the Bem Sex Role Inventory (7), sex role conservatism, religious involvement, time since the respondent became homosexually active, amount of time spent in the homosexual subculture, and relationship with father. Those who were most likely to become infected (independent of partner numbers) were more "masculine" (dominant and assertive) and less "feminine" (empathic and gentle) and were less likely to have religious involvement, to have become homosexually active fairly early in life, to spend a relatively high amount of time in the homosexual subculture, and to have had a relatively worse relationship with their father in adolescence. These findings permit a tentative psychological profile of the homosexual man most at risk of sexually transmitted disease infection.

The individual most at risk of infection is stereotypically "masculine" in his approach to sex, being a fairly assertive individual who is more likely to seek out partners actively than to wait to be approached. Such assertive masculinity, typical of the Mediterranean approach to sexuality in which the male's masculinity is measured in terms of his sexual prowess, is strikingly similar to what Silverstein (8) has referred to as "cult masculinity." Whether it has the driven quality of overcompensation or simply reflects a more active approach is a matter for conjecture at this stage. Silverstein suggests that cult masculinity *demands* sex with another person, and that the symbols of masculinity exert more pressure on behavior than the need for love. Of particular interest here is the observation by Silverstein that problems in homosexual men in dealing with love relationships are more likely to center around the father than the mother. Another variable, relationship with father, which is a predictor of number of times infected, is a striking empirical confirmation of this clinical observation. Psychodynamic interpretation would suggest that the man with the more negative relationship with his father is seeking to compensate by an overmasculine image and by seeking anonymous encounters in which risk of rejection by another male is minimized. It may also be the case that with each partner, the individual is seeking the acceptance from other males, implied in sexual gratification, that he was unable to obtain from his father, thus attempting to come to terms with paternal rejection by both masculine overcompensation and avoidance of intimacy.

Other variables which are predictors of a higher number of infections include religious involvement (the association of sex with sin and consequent guilt in most Christian denominations would be expected to lead to lower risk of infections), a longer time since becoming homosexually active (and thus a longer time the individual has to become infected), and the amount of leisure time spent in the homosexual subculture. This latter point does suggest that in those individuals most likely to become infected, their homosexuality has greater importance to them and is more strongly cathected. If this is the interpretation to be drawn from these data, it would suggest that where homosexuality is central to the individual's identity, there is a greater risk of infection through increased homosexual encounters. The picture that emerges of the individual at greatest risk of infection is thus of the masculine seeker of sex who may be reinforcing his identity and avoiding rejection from other males. The suggestion may be made that he also has difficulty in relating emotionally to other males as he had difficulty in relating to his father.

Confirmation of this view is provided if we look at the partner preferences of individuals in the four societies I studied, which predict increased infections of sexually transmitted diseases. The amount of variance of times infected which could be predicted by partner and respondent's own characteristics ranged from 48 percent (Australia) to 94 percent (Sweden). In other words, between half and nearly all of the variance in number of sexually transmitted diseases contracted could be accounted for by the preferred partners and the subject's own characteristics. Of the list of 18 characteristics with which respondents could rate themselves and their ideal partner, three partner characteristics (cold, masculine, and unconventional) and two self characteristics (extroverted and not hairy) predicted across more than one of the four countries. Three other salient characteristics noted for self or partner which also predicted across countries were the variables of genital size, sexiness, and height.

This adds to the picture of the homosexual man who is most likely to become infected with a sexually transmitted disease: he prefers partners who are emotionally cold, masculine, and somewhat unconventional. Such partners not only represent individuals with whom it is likely to be impossible to develop an emotional relationship, but also partners who appear to be followers of the same "cult masculinity": there is no chance of involvement, and the individual's own self-esteem and masculinity are probably bolstered by attracting such a partner. The individual's perception of himself as extroverted and with a smooth body suggests a degree of assertiveness and positive body image, which agree with previous theorizing about the homosexual man with high infection rates. It is also of interest that the other characteristics of concern for both partners and self were sexiness, penis size, and height; preoccupation with physical characteristics would appear to be related to perceptions of self and partner in those most at risk. Such findings point to a common underlying psychological process in homosexuals who are most likely to present with large numbers of previous sexually transmitted diseases, and it is precisely these individuals who appear to be most at risk of contracting AIDS as a sexually transmitted disease.

Turning to predictors of individuals who are most likely to have large numbers of partners, a second risk factor for AIDS, data on the same four societies reveal both complementary and discrepant variables. As for psychological predictors of larger numbers of infections, larger numbers of partners are again predicted by masculinity, reinforcing the suggestion that cult masculinity is associated with frequent sexual conquests. Apart from this, however, the data (fully described elsewhere [6]) reveal different predictors for relative promiscuity. The suggestion that different psychological factors are involved in relative promiscuity and numbers of infections thus appears to be born out by these data: the additional variables include educational level, age, position on the Kinsey Scale (degree of homosexuality or heterosexuality), expected societal reactions to one's homosexuality, and relationship with mother during adolescence.

From these data, then, the best predictors of high partner numbers (accounting for between 16 percent and 28 percent of its variance) are increased masculinity (referred to previously), lower level of education, older age, considering oneself more bisexual, expecting a more negative reaction to one's homosexuality from significant others and from society in general, and a worse relationship with mother during adolescence. Again, a psychodynamically coherent picture of such an individual is not hard to produce. What, then, motivates the homosexual man who has relatively large partner numbers?

In addition to noting that in no case did the number of infections associate with high partner numbers, the relatively promiscuous are older, which may imply a need to build up self-esteem and a sense of still being a desirable partner as the individual ages. Possibly, given the association with lower education and an expected negative reaction to homosexuality by society and acquaintances, the higher numbers of partners also serve to differentiate the individual who wishes to avoid close emotional homosexual or homosocial ties from those who tend to limit themselves to fewer, and possibly longer lasting, contacts. Of central interest, however, is the fact that those relatively more promiscuous homosexuals also describe themselves as more bisexual (or deny that they are exclusively homosexual). Tied in with the expectation of a more negative reaction to homosexuality, these data strongly suggest a degree of denial or unhappiness with homosexuality which is manifest in an inability or unwillingness to develop longer-term contacts. Such an inability or unwillingness would be a result of denial that one was "really homosexual," and thus had sexual contacts for sexual rather than emotional gratification, and an unwillingness to reveal one's sexual orientation by having steadier contacts which might make one's orientation more obvious to others. More likely, however, is the possibility that any form of homosexual commitment would either challenge the defense of bisexuality, or that it would be incompatible with the individual's idea that homosexuality is somewhat negative and that commitment is therefore incompatible with guilt-engendering sexual activity.

Finally, there is the involvement of psychodynamic factors in the association of a poor relationship with the mother during adolescence, and relative promiscuity. This is quite the opposite of the poor relationship with the *father*, which was found to predict high infections and, presumably, high degree of anonymous sex. However, it is particularly interesting that Šípová and Brzek (9) report that homosexual men model their behavior towards their partners' on their mother's behavior rather than their father's behavior and that the more effeminate they were, the more their partner-self behavior (in terms of love-hostility and dominance-submission) was like that of their mother. These results strongly suggest that a negative relationship with the mother is a model for future partner behavior, and that the association between a poor relationship with mother and relative promiscuity is not coincidental; the association is between a poor relationship model in adolescence and inability to relate to homosexual partners in later life. A lack of ability to accept one's sexual orientation at a social and emotional (though not a sexual) level also appears to predispose to larger numbers of partners. Again, the implications of this for AIDS infection are clear: large numbers of partners appear to be a second major risk factor in contracting AIDS sexually.

How much of the psychodynamics of sexually transmitted diseases fits with what is known of the epidemiology of AIDS cases? Jaffe et al. (3) noted that the best epidemiological predictors of AIDS included Italian, Jewish, or eastern European ancestry; previous sexually transmitted diseases; sexual activity (particularly feces exposure and rectal trauma scores); whether individuals had been heterosexually married; and most important, number of sex partners and proportion of partners from bathhouses (anonymous sex) as well as age of becoming homosexually active. The degree of fit of all these variables with the predictors of both number of infections and number of partners is good. First, the variable of Mediterranean or eastern European ancestry, while almost certainly linked with increased HLA-DR5 antigen frequency, may also be associated with the Mediterranean sexual style in which masculinity is defined in terms of number of sexual conquests, and thus also acts as a marker for a particular behavioral style of sexual gratification. Second, the association of previous marriage with AIDS cases fits the psychodynamic theory well. In an extensive analysis of married homosexual men (10), I noted that the best predictor of heterosexual marriage in homosexual men is an expectation of negative reaction to their homosexuality and a denial of the degree of their homosexuality. Thus, the link between a lack of comfort with one's homosexuality and higher partner numbers appears to be confirmed by an independent investigation of a U.S. population.

While there is a fair degree of internal consistency within the data presented here, which is supported by other investigations into psychological aspects of homosexuality as well as epidemiological investigations of homosexual AIDS cases, the psychovenereology of AIDS has not been specifically examined to date, and these conclusions must be regarded as tentative unless empirically and clinically confirmed. Nevertheless, they do offer a number of testable hypotheses from which further study may be generated; at this stage, it may be appropriate to present an outline of the probable psychovenereology of AIDS.

Two general dynamics, probably to some degree independent of one another, appear to be operating; the factors they influence are probably anonymity of partner and number of partners. AIDS cases to date would appear to be high on both. High partner anonymity appears to be associated with "cult masculinity," becoming homosexually active fairly early in life, lack of religious involvement, and a poor relationship with the father in adolescence, which may lead to individuals attempting to come to terms with paternal rejection by sexual contact with desirable males while avoiding the risk of rejection.

High partner numbers appear to share a similar dynamic in terms of "cult masculinity," but from this differ markedly. Those with higher partner numbers appear to be older and perhaps attempting to maintain self-esteem by way of convincing themselves of continuing sexual desirability. However, those with higher partner numbers appear also to expect more negative reactions to their homosexuality from society, and to deny the degree of their homosexual involvement. To such individuals, higher partner numbers probably represent an inability to accept their homosexuality as an emotional orientation to other males rather than as a form of sexual release, which they are less committed to by being "bisexual." Added to this, the lack of a satisfactory relationship with their mothers in adolescence appears to be consistent with the lack of an adequate model from which homosocial, as well as homosexual, behavior towards a partner may be derived.

Nevertheless, there is still an urgent need for a general psychosocial or psychodynamic model of determinants of sexual behavior in the male homosexual. It is still not clear whether increased partner numbers in general represent an attempt to increase self-esteem by constant validation of one's worth as a sexual partner, or represent a hedonistic acceptance of one's homosexuality. It may be possible to test this by assessing whether AIDS patients, with imposed celibacy, decompensate on being unable to continue sex, or increase autoerotic activity in compensation. Unfortunately, the trauma of suffering from a potentially terminal illness may obscure such reactions. From the data already presented, it is probable that there is a point beyond which high partner numbers and high level of anonymity in sex may be indicative of decreased psychological comfort, while at much lower levels it may be indicative of increased acceptance of one's sexual orientation, in a U-shaped curve. Whatever the findings, it is clear that psychovenereology has something to offer in terms of understanding risk factors in sexually transmitted diseases and AIDS in particular.

While I have attempted to outline some of the possible psychosocial and psychodynamic factors which contribute to the behaviors which put homosexuals most at risk of contracting AIDS, it is still an open question whether any psychological interventions may modify these. Further research, particularly on the effects of psychological factors on immune competence and the possibility of some individuals being more susceptible to infection than others as a result of psychological pressures, is needed. However, the fact that psychosocial factors are a better predictor of number of infections with sexually transmitted diseases in homosexual men than partner numbers does reinforce the fact that psychovenereology has a role in the understanding of the factors which predispose to AIDS infection.

References

1. Pinching AJ, McManus TJ, Jeffries DJ, et al: Studies of cellular immunity in male homosexuals in London. Lancet 2:126–130, 1983

2. Ader R: Behavioral influences on immune responses, Perspectives on Behavioral Medicine. Edited by Weiss SM, Herd JA, Fox BH. New York; Academic Press, 1981, p 163–182

3. Jaffe HW, Choi K, Thomas PA, et al: National case-control study of Kaposi's sarcoma and *Pneumocystis carinii* pneumonia in homosexual men, I: epidemiologic results. Ann Intern Med 99:145–151, 1983

4. Ross MW: Sexually transmitted diseases in homosexual men: a study of four societies. Br J Vener Dis (in press)

5. Ross MW: Socio-psychological predictors of STD infection in homosexual men: a study of four countries. Br J Vener Dis (in press)

6. Ross MW: Predictors of partner numbers in homosexual men: psychosocial factors in four societies. Sex Transm Dis (in press)

7. Bem SL: The measurement of psychological androgyny. J Consult Clin Psychol 42:155–162, 1974

8. Silverstein C: Man to Man: Gay Couples in America. New York, William Morrow, 1981

9. Šípová I, Brzek A: Parental and interpersonal relationships of transsexual and masculine and feminine homosexual men. J Homosex 9:75–85, 1983

12

Mental Health Aspects of Acquired Immune Deficiency Syndrome: Priorities for Research

Harold Alan Pincus, M.D.

12

Mental Health Aspects of Acquired Immune Deficiency Syndrome: Priorities for Research

The acquired immune deficiency syndrome (AIDS) has been given the federal government's highest priority for emergency health problems. To date, few published reports of AIDS take note of the behavioral and psychosocial reactions associated with this syndrome (1). The perspectives offered throughout this monograph, however, make resoundingly evident the significance of mental health issues in relation to AIDS. These issues arise both from the pathophysiology of the disease and its sequelae as well as from the special psychological implications of the syndrome and its sociocultural context. Moreover, these implications range far beyond the AIDS patients themselves, affecting those at high risk for the disorder, family members, lovers, friends, health care workers, and the public.

The interrelationship between biological and behavioral variables is increasingly recognized as a major frontier for health research. The recent report of the Institute of Medicine of the National Academy of Sciences on "Health and Behavior: Frontiers of Research in the Biobehavioral Sciences" demonstrates the relevance of these issues for health promotion and disease prevention. It also describes some of the many promising research opportunities in the interface between health and behavior (2). Research on the psychiatric and behavioral aspects of AIDS can serve as an important paradigm for this kind of biobehavioral investigation. Studies on the co-occurrence of psychiatric and medical disorders are important to advancing the science base of consultation-liaison psychiatry, primary care, and specialty medicine. Furthermore, the new clinical approaches to AIDS, which are developed in response to its mental health aspects, can serve as important models in planning interventions in other catastrophic health emergencies that affect large segments of the population.

The development and support of research in these areas has been a major interest to the Alcohol, Drug Abuse, and Mental Health Administration and its institutes, the National Institute of Mental Health, the National Institute of Drug Abuse, and the National Institute on Alcohol Abuse and Alcoholism. Research efforts are being made on a number of levels: initiating intramural research at the Clinical Center of the National Institutes of Health, encouraging individual investigators to develop research grant applications, and coordinating efforts with the various NIH institutes. Substantively, the areas of needed research cut across the full range of the scientific fields of epidemiology, the basic neurosciences, the behavioral sciences, clinical research, and treatment and prevention research.

Research is needed to clarify 1) the behavioral factors which might affect the etiopathogenesis and course of the disorder, 2) the behavioral consequences of the disorder, and 3) the utility of interventions to modify, treat, or prevent these behavioral processes and consequences. Studies within the first category are aimed at identifying psychological and behavioral factors, including drug abuse–related factors, which increase AIDS vulnerability in at-risk populations. For example, case control epidemiologic studies of intravenous drug abusers could gather basic information about the immune status of drug users as well as such lifestyle factors as nutrition, specific drug-taking behaviors, sanitary conditions, etc. to develop techniques for predicting the development of AIDS, and its specific course, in this group. Similar studies of behavioral factors with other risk groups are needed as are studies of the possible synergy between, for example, the particular homosexual lifestyle and intravenous drug use in predisposing an individual to AIDS. Psychoimmunologic and neuroendocrinologic studies are also needed to further investigate the effects of abused drugs, stress, and other biobehavioral factors on immune response.

The behavioral consequences of AIDS are far reaching, affecting not only people afflicted with the disease but also the members of risk groups; the family members, friends, and lovers of people with AIDS; and health care providers. AIDS patients may develop both primary and secondary mental symptoms. The relatively high prevalence of organic mental syndromes found among them, generally from an infectious etiology, needs to be studied to define the etiology and course of disease development, to identify more specific factors which place people at risk for AIDS, and to characterize discrete syndromes which will assist in the differential diagnosis. Secondary mental health consequences (reactions to the disease process) of AIDS are virtually always significant and may include severe anxiety or depressive syndromes and even suicidal behavior.

Retrospective and prospective studies are needed which focus on psychosocial, behavioral, and neurobiological factors associated with the development of specific psychiatric disturbances in AIDS patients and in members of risk groups (including both the "worried well" and those with the possible presyndromal symptoms). Included in this area are risk-assessment studies to refine the procedures for determining those individuals with AIDS or in risk populations who are likely to experience emotional disturbance or psychological dysfunction and studies to examine the relationship between social, behavioral, and psychological factors to the course and prognosis of the illness.

Interventions aimed at reducing behaviors which may be linked to the transmission or development of AIDS, as well as those involved with the treatment or prevention of the mental health sequelae from the disease, need to be assessed in a rigorous manner. Such studies would promote more effective care for those affected by AIDS, and assist in the development of effective strategies for other, similar situations. Specific educational strategies for modifying risk-related behaviors of persons at risk should also be evaluated. The relative roles of various generic treatment approaches (such as stress prediction and counseling) and specific techniques (such as particular forms of psychiatry or support group systems such as the Gay Men's Health Crisis and the Shanti Project) for treating mental health syndromes manifested in AIDS patients should be assessed in terms of both reducing psychiatric symptoms as well as altering the course and progression of the illness itself. There is also a need for research assessing the effect of preventive interventions in reducing stress and the incidence of emotional disturbance and psychological dysfunction in persons affected by AIDS.

Finally, cutting across all of these research areas are important methodological issues that need to be addressed. That is, given the unique subcultural contexts of this syndrome, researchers will need to examine these issues within the perspective of the gay culture, the drug abuse culture, the Haitian culture, etc. in order to maximize validity. Methodological studies and the development of instruments sensitive to issues of response bias and response validity with regard to subcultural and related issues are critical.

References

1. Holtz H, Dobro J, Palinkas R, et al: Psychosocial impact of acquired immune deficiency syndrome. JAMA, 250:163, 1983

2. Institute of Medicine: Health and Behavior: Frontiers of Research in the Biobehavioral Sciences. Washington, DC, National Academy Press, 1982

Epilogue

Acquired Immune Deficiency Syndrome: The Challenge to Psychiatry

James P. Krajeski, M.D.

Epilogue

Acquired Immune Deficiency Syndrome: The Challenge to Psychiatry

A few years ago polio was a dreaded disease for which medical science could offer no solution. Even today we are plagued by forms of cancer which we are forced to accept as untreatable. One might argue that acquired immune deficiency syndrome (AIDS) is not unlike these diseases and that the role of psychiatry in responding to AIDS is essentially the same as it would be with any devastating illness. Yet this argument overlooks the point that AIDS strikes heavily among people who have already been stigmatized by our society. It is true that in some ways it is not unlike other life-threatening illnesses; however, it is made unique by specific medical, psychological, and social factors which complicate responses to it. For example, a community's reaction to AIDS may result as much from AIDS being tied to homosexuality in the public mind as it does from the nature of the disease. Because psychiatrists are trained both in medicine and in mental health, the psychiatrist is ideally qualified to tackle the challenge of this syndrome which involves an interplay of these diverse forces.

The most obvious role for the psychiatrist to assume is the typical one of providing direct, individual care. This service may be aimed at a spectrum of individuals ranging from the "worried well" to persons with AIDS, and is discussed thoroughly in this monograph. Family therapy is another standard treatment modality that psychiatrists may offer which involves direct patient care. However, it may require some innovations such as a broadening of traditional concepts of family to include lovers and close friends. In working with families, a major focus of therapy may be the acceptance or rejection of persons with AIDS by family members. Families may also require assistance to deal with new information about a family member, for example, learning that someone is gay and has a life-threatening illness.

The psychiatrist also has a role in facilitating a team approach in treating the person with AIDS. The patient may require a variety of services, including medical, psychological, social, and spiritual ones, which involve many health care providers and other individuals. It is essential that all members of the treatment team interact smoothly to provide good care. However, the multitude of uncertainties about AIDS may encourage a splintering of opinions and treatment approaches. The psychiatrist may, at times, have to serve as a mediator to ensure that all team members respond in a coordinated, helpful manner.

Patients may be devastated by the effects of disease and may be physically and psychologically unable to look out for their best interests. In this case, psychiatrists should appropriately serve as advocates for their patients to see that appropriate medical care is given and that inappropriate care or restrictions are avoided. For example, in establishing medical protocols to be used in treating AIDS patients, there is a danger that isolation procedures may be developed which may not be medically warranted as the result of unreasonable fears of staff with insufficient regard for the psychological consequences to the patient. The psychiatrist must be able to assist involved staff to examine the motivation for their actions and to distinguish reasonable actions from unreasonable ones.

Still another challenge for the psychiatrist is that of meeting the mental health needs of health care workers and others who are directly involved in caring for persons with AIDS. The day-to-day care of terminally ill patients carries with it a significant element of stress. If physicians and others see their role primarily as one of "saving lives," they may suffer because of their ineffectiveness. However, if they can view their role in a broader sense of ministering to the ill or dying, they may be better able to cope with their expectations. The lack of certainty of the mode of transmission of AIDS may place stress on those who deal directly with the individual with AIDS, even though there is no evidence to suggest that AIDS has been transmitted to health care workers in the course of their work. Certain categories of individuals such as gay health care workers may face additional stress by virtue of belonging to a "risk" group and being faced on a regular basis with the human vulnerability to illness and death. The psychiatrist should be instrumental in addressing the emotional needs of this group as they carry out the important duties of their professions.

Psychiatry's role as described to this point involves traditional concepts of intervention and treatment of those affected directly or indirectly by AIDS. In looking at other roles for psychiatry, one recognizes that the major obstacle in combating AIDS is the lack of knowledge about the syndrome. Following the recent identification of the putative agent responsible for AIDS, ongoing research to delineate the role of HTLV III and to develop effective measures for prevention and treatment is a goal of all those concerned about AIDS. It is important that the voice of psychiatry be heard regarding research design and research funding. It is important to ensure that research into the psychological aspects of AIDS both with regard to prevention and treatment be adequately addressed. Studies are needed regarding the influence of psychological factors on immune system function. Research is necessary to determine how the psychological needs of all those involved in the AIDS crises can best be met. Research on prejudice and its ramifications in contributing to illness or interfering with the treatment of illness is warranted. There also exists a need for further exploration of aspects of human sexuality, particularly research which will assist in overcoming prejudice related to sexuality. Ultimately, in this area science should be able to help us to separate fact from fantasy or prejudice.

Psychiatry already has a considerable body of knowledge regarding prejudice and its effects. One challenge to psychiatry is to assist society to assess, understand, and accept differences among human beings and to identify and label prejudice where it exists. Certainly the treatment of the medical and psychiatric consequences of AIDS as well as aspects of prevention of AIDS are complicated by society's condemnation of certain groups of people. One of these stigmatized groups, namely gay men, will serve as an example for discussion purposes, but the role of psychiatry may be quite similar with other stigmatized groups.

Stigmatization of gay men has resulted in an atmosphere in which even a medical journal published editorial remarks by a minister suggesting that AIDS may be divine punishment for transgression of "universal natural moral law" (1). Were there not a general climate in our society which unthinkingly accepts such prejudicial judgments against stigmatized groups, we would not see such attitudes fostered in public. One could imagine the justifiable outcry that would follow if one were to suggest that breast cancer is a punishment for women's transgression of "universal natural moral law" or that sickle cell disease is a punishment for blacks' transgressions. In the past, psychiatry played a role in stigmatizing homosexuality by labelling it as an illness. Such a label gave fuel to those who were opposed to homosexuality on other grounds. So even though psychiatry no longer considers homosexuality as a mental illness, such concepts continue to be used by those who would discriminate against gay people. Without such arguments, people would often be faced with their own prejudice against individuals whom they do not really know or understand.

Facing a fatal and mysterious illness such as AIDS is a horrendous task. Facing the same circumstances as a member of a stigmatized group is even worse, if one can then be blamed for one's illness or one can be viewed as deserving of the illness. Prejudice can subtly influence judgments about funding and treatment decisions. Prejudice can create turmoil for families who are faced with the knowledge that a family member belongs to a stigmatized group. Worse yet, prejudice can be incorporated by the person with AIDS, and one can spend the last days of one's life tormented by self-hatred, remorse, and a feeling that one deserves retribution. Making peace with oneself and the world may become impossible.

Psychiatry's role in combating the disastrous mental health effects of prejudice is a challenging one. Prejudice is not something that when pointed out is like a piece of stained clothing which can be easily seen by the wearer, removed, and laundered. More often prejudice is not recognized as such; it is deeply ingrained and therefore cannot easily be identified and discarded or changed. Yet, one must begin somewhere, and psychiatry can help people to accept diversity as natural and strengthening to society as a whole. Psychiatry as a discipline which studies human behavior can educate health care providers and the public about gay people; it can help to explain and interpret the behavior of people involved in the AIDS crises; and it can point out the mental and physical consequences of prejudice.

In this role psychiatrists can help the gay individual to overcome internalized homophobia. They can aid the medical community by making certain that negative stereotypes which interfere with the provision of appropriate medical and psychological care are challenged and corrected. They can assist in sorting out rational responses from irrational ones. To accomplish this psychiatrists may need to provide general education that dispels the frequent misperception that all gay people are the same or that gay people are markedly different from heterosexuals.

Psychiatry may be particularly helpful in dealing with the public response to the AIDS crises. It is understandable that people will become anxious when faced with a condition that is life-threatening and for which there is limited information. But even in this circumstance there is appropriate and inappropriate anxiety. There is appropriate and inappropriate action. It is important that psychiatrists help society to deal rationally with AIDS and that psychiatry work to limit panic and other irrational responses. Here, too, psychiatrists can help to untangle and clarify those actions which are derived from prejudice or ignorance from actions which are responsible. Psychiatrists also have a role in preventing a polarization of society into "them" against "us," with the "them" being a stigmatized group. These groups may then be viewed as the enemy who is responsible for this condition. In fact many members, if not most members, of the so-called "high risk groups" are at no greater risk than the general society.

There has been considerable controversy over the adequacy of the government's funding for research and the adequacy of government efforts to combat AIDS. It has been alleged that because the groups of people most affected by AIDS have been viewed by many as societal outcasts, the government's response has been slow and inadequate compared to the response one would expect if a more "mainstream" group had been affected. Psychiatry, with its dual expertise involving both physical and mental health, can provide ideal consultants to political entities and public agencies to assist in developing reasonable and expedient public policies and to avoid policy-making on the basis of bias or a lack of medical/psychological knowledge. As more individuals are directly affected and aware of the impact of AIDS, there will be an increased need by governmental agencies, courts, and legislatures for sound psychiatric advice so that they can respond in a way which will avoid public panic and will be truly helpful in combating the physical and mental effects of this disease.

Prevention of AIDS is another area in which psychiatry should involve itself. Prevention is directly linked to whether or not individuals follow guidelines designed to limit the transmission of the disease. However, there are a number of reasons involving psychological subtleties which explain why some individuals may ignore established guidelines. It may be difficult for members of stigmatized groups to trust that "experts" are really providing reliable and bias-free information. Some suggestions may be disregarded if they are seen as based on bias rather than on reasonable scientific data. For example, gay men may reject advice which tells them to stop certain sexual practices if they feel that the advice-giver is really espousing concepts of morality rather than sound scientific principles. It would be important to utilize psychiatric consultation to determine how best to disseminate information so that it will be accepted by and meaningful to the intended recipients.

Stigmatization of group members may also result in behaviors which are conducive to the transmission of AIDS. For example, anonymous sexual activities in which one knows nothing of the health of one's partner may be a risk factor in AIDS. However, if one keeps sexual orientation a secret for fear of societal recriminations, one may be more prone to engage in relatively anonymous encounters where the risk of public identification is less. If psychiatry can meet the challenge of removing an unwarranted stigma, efforts at prevention may be more effective. Also if, as many assume, there is a relationship between immune function and stress, then reducing stress by removing stigma might also assist in prevention.

If these are roles that psychiatrists should play during this AIDS crisis, how can they best carry out their work? In many cases the individual practitioner will be in the best position to take action, for example, in treating individual patients and families or in developing local consultation and liaison services. However, some of the roles of psychiatry will require coordination and action through professional organizations at a national level. The American Psychiatric Association would be well suited to handle many of the issues concerning public education, research assessment, political action, health care funding, and the removal of stigmatization. In fact, the APA is in the process of fulfilling its legitimate role.

It is important, however, that AIDS not be considered as the problem of a particular group—e.g., a "gay" problem. Even if certain populations are affected in a disproportionate manner, AIDS is a health problem which touches on the lives of virtually everyone in some way. Dealing with this problem should properly involve the expertise of multiple APA committees and components. The APA should be prepared to coordinate its efforts with other groups who are working to combat AIDS including self-help groups, national foundations and organizations, and specialized professional groups such as gay physicians organizations. A special effort should be made to include and encourage participation by APA members who may have special expertise or interest in AIDS, such as gay psychiatrists and psychiatrists who have gay patients.

These efforts at delineating the role of psychiatry in the AIDS crisis are preliminary ones. As our knowledge of AIDS increases, the role of psychiatry may be expected to change. Even with our limited understanding of this devastating syndrome, we have the capability of treating, educating, consulting, and alleviating suffering. We can teach people to be compassionate, understanding, and accepting of diversity in our society. We can help people to put aside prejudice and to kindle a spark of kindness and caring so that we may all experience ourselves as more meaningfully human. That is the ultimate challenge to psychiatry that AIDS has presented to us.

Reference

1. Selby GI: AIDS and the moral law. North Carolina Medical Journal 44:275, 1983